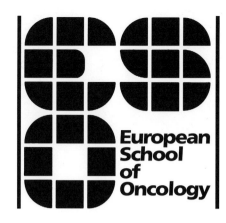

Monographs

Series Editor: U. Veronesi

The European School of Oncology gratefully acknowledges sponsorship for the Task Force received from  STERLING WINTHROP

P. Workman (Ed.)

New Approaches in Cancer Pharmacology: Drug Design and Development

With 24 Figures and 7 Tables

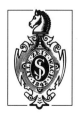
Springer-Verlag
Berlin Heidelberg New York
London Paris Tokyo
Hong Kong Barcelona
Budapest

Professor Paul Workman (Chairman and Editor)

Cancer Research Campaign Beatson Laboratories
CRC Department of Medical Oncology
University of Glasgow
Alexander Stone Building
Garscube Estate, Switchback Road
Bearsden, Glasgow G61 1BD, UK

Dr. Maurizio D'Incalci (Co-chairman)

Istituto Mario Negri
Via Eritrea 62
20157 Milano, Italy

ISBN 3-540-56089-0 Springer-Verlag Berlin Heidelberg New York
ISBN 0-387-56089-0 Springer-Verlag New York Berlin Heidelberg

Library of Congress Cataloging-in-Publication Data
New approaches in cancer pharmacology : drug design and development / Paul Workman (ed.).
  (Monographs /European School of Oncology)
Includes bibliographical references and index.
  ISBN 3-540-56089-0 (alk. paper)
  ISBN 0-387-56089-0 (alk. paper)
1. Antineoplastic agents. 2. Cancer-Gene therapy. 3. Biological response modifiers. 4. Cancer-Molecular aspects. I.
Workman, Paul. II. Series: Monographs (European School of Oncology) [DNLM: 1. Antineoplastic Agents-pharmacology.
2. Drug Design. QV 269 N53167] RC271.C5N43 1992 616.99'4061–dc20 DNLM/DLC for Library of Congress

Typesetting: Camera ready by editor
Printing: Druckhaus Beltz, Hemsbach/Bergstr.; Binding: J. Schäffer GmbH & Co. KG, Grünstadt
23/3145 - 5 4 3 2 1 0 - Printed on acid-free paper

Foreword

The European School of Oncology came into existence to respond to a need for information, education and training in the field of the diagnosis and treatment of cancer. There are two main reasons why such an initiative was considered necessary. Firstly, the teaching of oncology requires a rigorously multidisciplinary approach which is difficult for the Universities to put into practice since their system is mainly disciplinary orientated. Secondly, the rate of technological development that impinges on the diagnosis and treatment of cancer has been so rapid that it is not an easy task for medical faculties to adapt their curricula flexibly.

With its residential courses for organ pathologies and the seminars on new techniques (laser, monoclonal antibodies, imaging techniques etc.) or on the principal therapeutic controversies (conservative or mutilating surgery, primary or adjuvant chemotherapy, radiotherapy alone or integrated), it is the ambition of the European School of Oncology to fill a cultural and scientific gap and, thereby, create a bridge between the University and Industry and between these two and daily medical practice.

One of the more recent initiatives of ESO has been the institution of permanent study groups, also called task forces, where a limited number of leading experts are invited to meet once a year with the aim of defining the state of the art and possibly reaching a consensus on future developments in specific fields of oncology.

The ESO Monograph series was designed with the specific purpose of disseminating the results of these study group meetings, and providing concise and updated reviews of the topic discussed.

It was decided to keep the layout relatively simple, in order to restrict the costs and make the monographs available in the shortest possible time, thus overcoming a common problem in medical literature: that of the material being outdated even before publication.

UMBERTO VERONESI
Chairman Scientific Committee
European School of Oncology

Contents

Introduction

Paul Workman

Cancer Research Campaign Beatson Laboratories, CRC Department of Medical Oncology, University of Glasgow, Alexander Stone Building, Garscube Estate, Switchback Road, Bearsden, Glasgow G61 1BD, United Kingdom

Cancer pharmacology is now a highly sophisticated business. Never really part of mainstream pharmacology, it is based traditionally in the specialist cancer institutes and its main focus has been the rational design and development of new anticancer drugs and the understanding and optimal use of existing agents.

The techniques now available to cancer pharmacologists are infinitely more powerful than ever before and the standards required throughout the drug development process have quite rightly become increasingly more demanding. Particularly striking has been the exhilarating pace at which our comprehension of the molecular basis of the cancer cell has expanded, coupled with access to the methodologies and reagents of recombinant DNA technology.

We cannot yet design a drug from first principles. Nevertheless, the design element is undoubtedly increasing and the drug development process is becoming progressively ever more rational. Most of our existing agents interact directly with DNA synthesis and the associated mechanics of cell replication. Many workers feel that drugs of this type can be optimised by rational means and new molecular techniques. Equally well, others argue that we should seek out new targets for the development of cancer drugs, particularly among the changes in oncogenes and tumour suppressor genes that are increasingly found to drive the malignant phenotype of cancer cells.

Our Task Force was created to examine progress and predict future trends in cancer pharmacology generally, and in drug design and development in particular. A large number of topics could have been covered and we have had to be selective for reasons of space.

This first Monograph opens with a review by Maurizio D'Incalci (Milano) of DNA sequence and gene-specific drugs. The important impact of molecular biology techniques is very well illustrated here. The ability to define in remarkable detail the precise molecular interactions of DNA-interactive drugs is clearly shown. Also emphasised are the prospects for improving on sequence specificity with CC-1065, distamycin mustard and related agents, some of which are now in clinical trial. However, even the best sequence-specific DNA-interactive chemical can recognise no more than a 5-6 base pair sequence. By contrast, Claude Hélène (Paris) illustrates the much greater molecular recognition capability of antisense and antigene oligonucleotides. Mutant *ras* genes can be distinguished from the normal counterpart and growth inhibition of oncogenic *ras*-transformed cells *in vitro* can be achieved. Here the difficulties concern the pharmacokinetic aspects - particularly uptake into cells in solid tumours.

Moving one step further, Karol Sikora (Hammersmith) assesses prospects for biological and gene therapies. The limitations of the cytokines in current use are mentioned and the exciting if futuristic possibilities of gene therapy are stressed. Sikora is also positive about the potential of interfering with signal transduction pathways in cancer cells, a theme subsequently taken up by John Hickman (Manchester). While supporting these approaches to antagonising the growth-promoting effects of oncogenes and growth factors, Hickman is careful to point out the drawbacks of focusing exclusively on mitogenic signalling pathways, such as those driven by the epidermal growth factor receptor. We are reminded of our relative ignorance of the transduction pathways involved in differentiation and programmed cell death (or apoptosis) and of the signal cascades which dictate responses to cellular damage - all potential new targets for therapy.

The development of endocrine agents has been a success story for the rational medicinal chemistry approach, and this area is summarized for us by Mike Jarman (Sutton). A new generation of antiendocrine agents is envisaged, with increasing input from modelling and computational chemistry - a development which is anticipated in all areas of anticancer drug development, but is not truly with us yet in reality. The presence of hypoxic cells in solid tumours is arguably the only physiological feature which differentiates them from normal tissues. Paul Workman (Glasgow) reviews current progress in the development of bioreductive agents which are activated selectively to toxic metabolites in hypoxic tumour cells. A new approach which is emphasised is the potential for optimising bioreductive drug structure to suit the catalytic preferences of enzymes that are hyperexpressed in cancers compared to normal tissues - for example DT-diaphorase - thus introducing a second level of solid-tumour selectivity. Workman stresses the importance of carrying out mechanistic studies not only in the preclinical work-up of a new drug, but also in the early clinical phase. This is very much in keeping with the contribution by Merril Egorin (Baltimore) who assesses the present status of therapeutic drug monitoring and dose optimisation in oncology. He reviews the theoretical and experimental basis for these approaches, and quotes a number of examples in which toxicity can be minimised and therapeutic effect maximised in individual patients. This is essential in a disease where the therapeutic index of our drugs is always likely to be limited.

Finally, Gilberto Schwartsmann (Amsterdam) deals with the controversial area of screening for antitumour drugs. Even as we search for better ways to design drugs on a rational basis, there remains a need to devise improved test systems which take into account the particular molecular target of interest, together with the relevant biology of human tumours. Schwartsmann is careful to point out that we will be looking increasingly to novel molecules developed by mechanism-based design to exploit known biological features and peculiarities of tumours. At the same time he reminds us that the current crop of agents which exhibit highly promising activity in early clinical studies - the antitubulin drugs taxol, taxotere and rhizoxin; the topoisomerase I inhibitors topotecan and CPT 11; and the DNA intercalating and topoisomerase II inhibitor DuP 941 - all hit more or less conventional molecular targets and were identified by traditional screening techniques. We can look at this in two ways. One is to accept that this success vindicates the traditional screening approach to cancer drug development. The other is more cautious - suggesting that perhaps we will run into similar problems with these agents as have befallen their predecessors acting on identical targets.

There are clearly different ways to proceed in the rational design and development of new anticancer drugs and yet there is probably still a place for random screening. Spectacular advances have been made in defining novel targets and harnessing new technologies to exploit these discoveries. We predict that the next decade will be a very exciting one for cancer pharmacology.

Acknowledgement

First of all, I thank my Task Force members for their time and enthusiastic commitment to the project. On behalf of them, I would like to thank the members of the European School of Oncology for their help: especially Vlatka Majstorovic for highly efficient organisation and Marije de Jager for painstaking and patient editorial support. Margaret Jenkins in Glasgow provided invaluable coordination skills. The city of Venice was as ever the perfect setting. Finally, I thank Sterling Winthrop for their generous support of this Task Force.

Sequence and Gene-Specific Drugs

Maurizio D'Incalci [1], Massimo Broggini [1] and John A. Hartley [2]

1   Istituto di Ricerche Farmacologiche Mario Negri, Via Eritrea 62, 20157 Milano, Italy
2   Department of Oncology, University College and Middlesex School of Medicine, 91 Riding House Street, London, United Kingdom

Several DNA interacting agents of diverse chemical structure are among the most clinically useful antineoplastic drugs. Although they are also toxic to normal tissues, they possess some degree of selectivity and specificity against a variety of human tumours. There are tumours which are particularly sensitive to DNA-interacting agents (e.g. testicular tumours are often curable with cisplatin), but the reasons for this peculiar sensitivity are still unclear. A better understanding of the molecular basis of the sensitivity to such agents is necessary before any attempt can be made to design molecules which are more selective for different types of human neoplasms.

The rapidly growing knowledge of tumour biology, coupled with the use of novel molecular biology and pharmacology techniques, make it possible to envisage experimental systems which could test precise hypotheses concerning the mechanisms of sensitivity and resistance to antineoplastic agents. In this chapter we will review some relevant aspects of the DNA sequence specificity of alkylating agents with different structures, and the effect of sequence-specific DNA damage on the regulation of gene transcription, stressing the potential importance of the application of new molecular pharmacology methods to the selection and investigation of novel drugs.

DNA Sequence-Specific Binding of Alkylating Agents Used in Cancer Chemotherapy

Methods have been available for several years to investigate DNA damage in total genomic DNA (e.g. single and double strand breaks, DNA-DNA interstrand crosslinks, DNA-protein-crosslinks) or to quantitate specific adducts on DNA bases. It has been known for a long time that the major site of alkylation of most alkylating agents currently used as chemotherapeutic agents is at the guanine N7 position with lesser reaction at guanine O6 and adenine N3. However, the techniques used did not discriminate between the relative alkylation of a given base depending on the DNA sequence in which it was located. This may be very relevant since one possible way to increase the specificity of DNA damaging agents could be to increase the damage towards selected DNA sequences which are important for the abnormal proliferation of cancer cells. Recently, methods for the determination of the pattern of alkylation of guanine N7 or adenine N3 have been developed, thus making it possible to reevaluate existing alkylating agents. The most widely used method is a modified sequencing technique based on the principle that the alkylation can be converted to a strand cleavage either by hot piperidine in the case of guanine N7 alkylation or by elevated temperature in the case of adenine N3 alkylation. The method has been successfully applied to obtain information on the pattern of guanine N7 alkylation of several alkylating agents used in cancer chemotherapy (see the section on major groove binders) and to characterise the adenine N3 alkylations of new experimental chemotherapeutic agents which bind in the minor groove (see the section on minor groove binders). However, these methods have important limitations in that they do not allow the determination of alkylations which are not converted to DNA-strand breaks. For example, cisplatinum adducts on guanine N7 cannot be pinpointed using these procedures as they are not converted to DNA-breaks by piperidine and O6 guanine alkylations cannot be converted to DNA-strand breaks by this method. Several alternatives are under investigation in different laboratories. The sequence specificity of DNA covalent adducts can be evaluated using enzymes which are stopped by the presence of the adducts. The termination of E. coli exonuclease III, E. coli polymerase [1] or the thermostable Taq DNA polymerase has been used to detect DNA sequence-specific damage of bifunctional alkylating agents and platinum (II) coordination complexes [2]. The Taq polymerase stop assay has the advantage that multiple cycles can increase sensitivity and has a potential use in intact cells exposed to the drugs at pharmacologically relevant concentrations. Some methods can be also applied to investigate the DNA sequence-specific interaction of drugs which bind DNA in a non-covalent manner. Of particular importance are footprinting assays, initially developed to investigate the DNA sequence-specific binding of proteins and then adapted to characterise the binding of smaller molecules. These techniques rely on the ability of ligands bound to DNA to protect DNA from the digestion of DNAse I [3] or radical producing chemicals (e.g. methidiiumpropyl-Fe-EDTA) [4]. The analysis of undigested DNA fragments by sequencing techniques gives information on the precise location and binding site size of the ligand on the DNA.

A number of papers describing the methods which are available for evaluating DNA sequence-specific binding of DNA-interacting agents, have recently been published [1,2,5,6]. Here we will give some examples of DNA sequence-specific interactions of anti-tumour agents which bind in the major and in the minor groove of DNA, stressing those aspects which are relevant for the design of new drugs. In addition, we will discuss the hypothesis that the antitumour activity of some DNA-interacting agents may be related to their ability to modify the recognition of transcription factors, thus causing impairment of the regulation of gene transcription. If this

can be verified it would lead to the possibility of investigating potential antitumour agents in a different way.

Major Groove Binders

Although nitrogen mustards are very toxic compounds they are still among the most effective agents for the therapy of some solid and haematological malignancies. It is unlikely that their relative selectivity simply relies on the greater growth rate of some sensitive tumours since the activity of these drugs is also demonstrated in a number of solid tumours which grow more slowly than other normal tissues. DNA is considered the most important target for the action of nitrogen mustards. It has been known for a long time that several DNA monoadducts and DNA-interstrand crosslinks are formed upon exposure of cells to nitrogen mustards. However, until recently very little was known about the precise location of nitrogen mustard-induced DNA lesions and it was believed that these highly reactive compounds did not possess any sequence-specific reaction with DNA. Recent studies have instead demonstrated that nitrogen mustards do not alkylate nucleophiles present in DNA in a random fashion. Important variations in the intensity of N7-guanine alkylations have been demonstrated among guanines in a DNA sequence following treatment with nitrogen mustards [6], chloroethylnitrosoureas [7] and alkyltriazenes [8]. Although differences exist in the preferential alkylation of various nitrogen mustards, it appears that their common feature is the much greater alkylation on guanines located within runs of contiguous guanines than on guanines located in other sequences. It has been shown that the intensity of alkylations correlates well with the calculated molecular electrostatic potential at the reactive site. The molecular electrostatic potential is sequence dependent and strongly influenced by its nearest neighbour base pairs [9]. Nevertheless, among some nitrogen mustards with different chemical structures there are distinct differences which are not related to their charge, but to the structure of their non-alkylating portion. For example, uracil mustard alkylates preferentially a guanine in the sequence 5'-pyrimidine G C, which is a weak alkylation site for most nitrogen mustards. It has been proposed that this peculiar sequence-specific alkylation is facilitated by the interaction between the uracil-O4 atom of the drug and the 3'-cytosine amino group. The reaction is favoured if the guanine is displaced towards its sugar-phosphate backbone as would occur when the guanine is situated between two pyrimidines [10].

In some cases the alkylation pattern of a parent compound may differ from that of the drug metabolite. This can occur even when the structural differences are small. For example, the sequence specificity of guanine N7 alkylation of dabis maleate differs from that of the uncharged hydrolysis product which was thought to be the ultimate alkylating species, thus suggesting that some still unidentified intermediate with a different sequence specificity for alkylation is formed [11]. Another example concerns the bioreductive alkylating agent 2,5-diaziridinyl-1,4-benzoquinone (DZQ). In contrast to all other diaziridinylbenzoquinones investigated which produced the same pattern of guanine-N7-alkylation as nitrogen mustards, DZQ when it is reduced to the hydroquinone form alkylates almost exclusively guanines located between a T and a C [12]. Therefore, hypoxic conditions may not only cause a quantitative increase in alkylation of DNA as occurs for all the diaziridinylbenzoquinones, but may modify the type of alkylation, becoming very selective for some specific sequences. This unique finding was explained by a model in which DZQ is intercalated between the guanine and the cytosine residues forming hydrogen bonding between the two hydroxyls of the hydroquinone and cytosine O2 and C4-NH2 groups, thus orienting the drug in an ideal position to alkylate the guanine N7 position in this sequence. This observation may be pharmacologically relevant considering that in most cases solid tumours have an inefficient vascularisation and therefore the oxygen tension is lower than in other normal tissues. If the peculiar sequence-specific alkylation of the hydroquinone has an antitumour effect, this should therefore be particularly marked in large advanced tumours than in better vascularised small neoplasms (see chapter by Workman, this volume).

The sequence specificity described for some alkylating agents has been essentially investigated with regard to N7 guanine monoalkylation. However, it is known that a much better antitumour effect can be achieved with bifunctional alkylating agents able to form crosslinks between two sites of DNA or between DNA and proteins. For some alkylators, such as nitrogen mustards or chloroethylnitrosoureas, a good correlation has been found between DNA-interstrand crosslinks and cytotoxicity [13]. Very little is known about the sequence specificity of DNA interstrand crosslink formation. It seems that the preferential crosslinks produced by nitrogen mustard does not occur in a 5'-GC sequence, as previously postulated, but rather in a 5'GNC sequence (where N = any base) [14]. It remains to be established, however, to what extent the different pattern of monoalkylation seen for nitrogen mustards with different substituents may influence the sequence specificity of the crosslinks. In the case of DZQ, however, it is clear that the unique specificity of the hydroquinone form of the drug results in a preferred crosslink at 5'-GC rather than the 5'GNC sequences seen for other diaziridinylbenzoquinones.

Minor Groove Binders

Among the available anticancer agents which are currently used in cancer chemotherapy only mitomycin C is known to bind covalently to DNA in the minor groove. In order to react with DNA, the drug undergoes a reduction of the quinone function and the reactive species alkylates the N2 position of guanine. The exact sequence specificity of the monoalkylation is a matter of some debate. However, the crosslinks are formed preferentially in 5'-CG sequences [15].

Two classes of recently developed minor groove alkylating agents are currently in initial clinical investigation. They are derivatives of the natural products CC-1065 and distamycin A, respectively, and their binding in the minor groove occurs in both cases at AT rich sequences. CC-1065 consists of 3 pyrrole indole subunits, one of which contains a DNA reactive cyclopropyl function. CC-1065 binds covalently to the N3 of adenines with a high degree of sequence specificity [16]. A preferential alkylation has been demonstrated for A located in the sequences 5'-AAAAA and 5'PuNTTA, where Pu represents either a G or A and N is any base.

Some derivatives such as carzelesin (U-80244) or adozelesin (U-73975) have been synthesised [17]. These are under initial clinical investigation due to their significant antitumour activity against rodent tumours and human xenografts and their improved therapeutic index compared to CC-1065.

Distamycin derivatives [18] contain alkylating moieties attached to the distamycin A molecule. The benzyl mustard derivative (FCE 24517) has shown marked sequence specificity for adenine alkylation [19] and it has good antitumour activity against rodent tumours and several human xenografts. In addition, it is not cross-resistant to other nitrogen mustards and it has been selected for phase I clinical trial, which is now in progress in Europe. The initial studies on the characterisation of the sequence-specific alkylation of adenine by CC-1065 and of the distamycin derivatives appear different; therefore these drugs could cause preferential damage on different gene sequences which may lead to different antitumour activity and toxicity profiles. It is still to be determined whether there is cross-resistance between different minor groove binders. Analogues of distamycin have been synthesised recently that recognise GC-containing sequences of increasing size in the minor groove, which may be useful in addressing some of these questions. In addition, it is now possible to rationally design sequence-specific minor groove crosslinking agents; for example, a highly active compound based on the pyrrolobenzodiazepine ring system has recently been synthesised which recognises 6 base pairs with a preference for 5'-PuGATCPy sequences, crosslinking between the 2 guanine-N2 positions [20].

Alteration of DNA Drug Binding and Impairment of the Function of Transcription Factors

The main mechanism of transcription regulation involves proteins which bind to regulatory elements of DNA in a sequence-specific manner, turning a gene on or off. DNA structure varies significantly when different DNA sequences are compared. According to the DNA sequence there are marked variations in the groove width, local twist and displacement of the average base pair plane to its neighbour. Small changes in these parameters can alter the specific recognition of regulatory proteins.

Recent work by this laboratory has shown that the binding of distamycin or distamycin derivatives to DNA can inhibit transcription factors which recognise specific AT-rich boxes [21]. The inhibition was found for factors such as OTF-1 which recognises the octamer ATTTGCAT but not for factors which recognise GC-rich DNA sequences. Recently, Dorn et al. [22] confirmed these findings using Antennapedia homeodomein (Antp HD) peptide or derivatives of a fushi tarazu homeodomain (ftz HD) peptide, which also have AT-rich binding sites. It is conceivable that this mechanism may be operative in many antineoplastic agents which bind to DNA with some degree of sequence specificity. We recently found that nitrogen mustard is able to inhibit the binding of transcription factors such as NFkB or sp1 to their GC-rich consensus sequences, but not of factors which bind to AT-rich sequences. It may be that the different spectrum of activity and the degree of selectivity of DNA-interacting agents is ultimately due to the selective inhibition of transcription of specific genes and one mechanism by which this may occur is the alteration of the specific recognition of transcription factors. We believe that, although the importance of these mechanisms for the antineoplastic activity of drugs is still to be demonstrated, it seems worthwhile to investigate the DNA-transcription factor complex as a potential target for chemotherapeutic agents. We believe that this approach merits particular attention for two main reasons. Firstly, an increased knowledge of the DNA sequence-specific binding of different compounds will make it possible to modify the local DNA sequence recognised by different DNA-binding proteins with much greater specificity. Secondly, current molecular biology research is producing new information on the mechanisms of regulation of transcription of different genes in different tissues, thus increasing the possibility of identifying suitable target factors.

Conclusions and Future Directions

Several compounds bind to DNA and cause DNA damage in a sequence-specific manner. We have described examples in which major or minor groove binders exhibit some degree of sequence specificity. Although far from being satisfactory, the degree of sequence specificity of alkylating agents currently used as antineoplastic agents is evident. It may be hypothesised that their relative selectivity against some tumours might be due in part to this specificity and that even small gains in specificity of base binding might lead to considerable increases in biological effect. Therefore, it seems worthwhile to develop new compounds with an enhanced or altered selectivity of damage to critical DNA sequences. In order to achieve this, further studies are required in several areas.

1. A critical question is whether the data that have been obtained on the sequence specificity of alkylation by incubating naked DNA *in vitro* with relatively high drug concentrations are representative of the pattern of sequence-specific DNA binding occurring in intact living cells, exposed to pharmacologically reasonable drug concentrations, and in tissues taken from animals or humans receiving tolerable drug doses.
This is obviously a very relevant question, the answer to which requires new and more sensitive assays which are under development in several laboratories. Preliminary studies from these laboratories indicate that for nitrogen mustards that give different sequence selectivities the patterns of alkylation are preserved in the highly reiterated human sequence of α-DNA in cells. If *in vitro* assays can reliably predict what happens in cells, then they can be used as a means to select compounds which are potentially interesting for future development. In addition, the definition of which lesions produced by a given drug are biologically the most important requires new methods of analysis. The most frequent sites of binding may not necessarily be the most biologically significant.

2. Another important question is: which are the DNA sequences to select as the most appropriate targets for human tumours? Sequences which are clearly responsible for the malignant behaviour of some haematological malignancies have been identified (see chapter by Hélène, this volume), but for most human tumours we still need a better characterisation of their molecular biology in order to select the appropriate target to obtain the maximum growth inhibitory and differentiating effect.

3. Of equal importance to the specificity of binding may be the specificity of repair of this binding, which may depend on the type of damage, the primary base sequence containing the damage, and the genomic location of the damage. In addition, the repair capacity of a particular DNA lesion may differ between different human tumour types.
Differential repair mechanisms could be relevant for the selectivity of action against certain tumours if it can be demonstrated that they are deficient for a critical repair mechanism.

4. If ultimately it was possible to develop a drug which is cytotoxic against a specific tumour cell because of its ability to cause a critical DNA lesion in a gene responsible for the malignant behaviour of that cell, it is likely that the clinical antitumour activity will be limited because human tumours are highly heterogeneous. This point is of course a limitation to any antitumour therapy addressed against a specific target. An approach utilising a combination of overlapping "specific therapies" may be required to produce a complete response.

5. The great advance in understanding the molecular biology of tumours that has been accomplished in the last decade has not been accompanied by an equivalent advance in the development of experimental systems to test the activity of potentially active antitumour agents. Molecules which are highly target specific should be tested against relevant experimental tumour systems. In this respect, we feel that it is realistic to obtain a significant improvement by either characterising existing systems (i.e., tumour cell lines, rodent tumours, human tumour xenografts) as much as possible for their biological properties (i.e.,

expression of different oncogenes, receptors of hormones and growth factors, DNA repair mechanisms, peculiar growth requirements, etc.), or setting up specific model systems (for example by the use of genetic manipulations) to verify the precise biological effect and therapeutic outcome of specific classes of drugs whose mechanism has been previously investigated *in vitro*.

We are confident that at least some of these areas will be elucidated in the near future, thereby increasing the chances of pursuing this approach in a more rational and successful way. Although the development of more DNA sequence-specific and gene-specific drugs is an exciting area of future work, many obstacles and difficulties lie ahead and an approach combining chemical, molecular and biological expertise will be required. Many clinically used anticancer agents were not rationally designed or have been designed on the basis of incorrect hypotheses; nevertheless, they have been effective in the therapy of some human malignancies. Hopefully the approaches we have described will generate rationally designed and superior DNA-interacting drugs for clinical development. These too may ultimately prove effective for unpredicted reasons, possibly related to the fact that a different way of selecting and investigating novel agents was used.

REFERENCES

1   Royer-Pokora B, Gordon LK and Haseltine WA: Use of exonuclease III to determine the site of stable lesions in defined sequences of DNA: the cyclobutane pyrimidine dimer and cis and trans dichlorodiammine platinum II examples. Nucleic Acids Res 1981 (9): 4595-4609

2   Ponti M, Forrow SM, Souhami RL, D'Incalci M and Hartley JA: Measurement of the sequence specificity of covalent DNA modification by antineoplastic agents using Taq DNA polymerase. Nucleic Acids Res 1991 (19): 2929-2933

3   Drew HR: Structural specificities of five commonly used DNA nucleases. J Molec Biology 1984 (176): 535-557

4   Dervan PB: Design of sequence-specific DNA-binding molecules. Science 1986 (232): 464-471

5   Raynolds VL, Molineux LJ, Kaplan D, Swenson DH and Hurley LH: Reaction of the antitumour antibiotic CC-1065 with DNA, location at the site of thermally induced strand breakage and analysis of DNA sequence specificity. Biochemistry 1985 (24): 6228-6237

6   Mattes WB, Harley JA and Kohn KW: DNA sequence selectivity of guanine N7 alkylation by nitrogen mustards. Nucleic Acids Res 1986 (14): 2971-2987

7   Hartley JA, Gibson NW, Kohn KW and Mattes WB: DNA sequence selectivity of guanine-N7 alkylation by three antitumour chlorethylating agents. Cancer Res 1986 (46): 1943-1947

8   Gibson NW, Mattes WB and Hartley JA: Identification of specific DNA lesions induced by three classes of chloroethylating agents: chloroethylnitrosoureas, chloroethylmethanesulfonates and chloroethylimidazotetrazines. Pharmac Ther 1985 (31): 153-163

9   Pullman A and Pullman B: Molecular electrostatic potential of the nucleic acids. Q Rev Biophys 1981 (14): 289-380

10 Kohn KW, Hartley JA and Mattes WB: Mechanisms of DNA seuqence selective alkylation of guanine-N7 positions by nitrogen mustards. Nucl Acids Res 1987 (14): 10531-10549

11 Broggini M, Hartley JA, Mattes WB, Ponti M, Kohn KW and D'Incalci M: DNA damage and sequence selectivity of DNA binding of the new anticancer agent 1,4-bis(2-Chloroethyl)-1,4-diazabicyclo-[2.2.1] heptane dimaleate. Br J Cancer 1990 (61): 285-289

12 Hartley JA, Berardini MD, Ponti M, Gibson NW, Thompson AS, Thurston DG, Hoey GM and Butler J: DNA crosslinking and sequence selectivity of aziridinylbenzoquinones: a unique reaction at 5'-GC-3' sequences with 3,6-diaziridinyl-1,4-benzoquinone upon reduction. Biochem 1991 (30): 11719-11724

13 Sunters A, Springer CJ, Coombes RC, Bagshawe K, Souhami RL and Hartley JA: A comparison between the cytotoxicity, DNA crosslinking ability, and DNA sequence selectivity of the aniline mustard derivatives melphalan, chlorambucil, and para-N-2(chloro-ethyl)benzoic acid. Biochem Pharmacol 1992 (41): in press

14 Hartley JA, Berardini MD and Souhami RL: An agarose gel method for the determination of DNA interstrand crosslinking applicable to the measurement of the rate of total and "second-arm" crosslink reactions. Analyt Biochem 1991 (193): 131-134

15 Borowy-Borowsky H, Lipman R, Chowdary D and Tomasz M: Recognition between mitomycin C and specific DNA sequences for crosslink formation. Biochemistry 1990 (29): 2999-3006

16 Hurley LH, Warpehoski MA, Lee CS, McGovern JP, Scahill TA, Kelly KC, Wicnieski NA, Gebhard I and Bradford VS: Sequence specificity of DNA alkylation by the unnatural enantiomers of CC-1065 and its synthetic analogs. J Am Chem Soc 1990 (112): 4633-4649

17 Li LH, Wallace TL, DeKoning TF, Warpehoski MA, Kelly RC, Priairie MD and Krueger WC: Structure and activity relationship of several novel CC-1065 analogs. Invest New Drugs 1987 (5): 329-337

18 Arcamone FM, Animati F, Barbieri B, Configliacchi E, D'Alessio R, Geroni C, Giuliani FC, Lazzari E, Menozzi M, Mongelli N, Penco S and Verini MA: Synthesis, DNA-binding properties, and antitumor activity of novel distamycin derivative. J Med Chem 1989 (32): 774-778

19 Broggini M, Erba E, Ponti M, Ballinari D, Geroni C, Spreafico F and D'Incalci M: Selective DNA interaction of the novel distamycin derivative FCE 24517. Cancer Res 1991 (51): 199-204

20 Bose DS, Thompson AS, Ching J, Hartley JA, Berardini MD, Jenkins TC, Neidle S, Hurley LH and Thurston DE: Rational design of a highly efficient irreversible DNA interstrand cross-linking agent based on the pyrrolobenzodiazepine ring system. J Am Chem Soc 1992 (114): 4939-4941

21 Broggini M, Ponti M, Ottolenghi S, D'Inalci M, Mongelli N and Mantovani R: Distamycins inhibit the binding of OTF-1 and NFE-1 transfactors to their conserved DNA elements. Nucleic Acids Res 1989 (17): 1051-1059

22 Dorn A, Affolter M, Müller M, Gehring WJ and Leupin W: Distamycin-induced inhibition of homeodomain-DNA complexes. EMBO J 1992 (11): 279-286

Antisense and Antigene Oligonucleotides Targeted to Oncogenes

Claude Hélène

Laboratoire de Biophysique, Muséum National d'Histoire Naturelle, INSERM U.201 - CNRS UA.481, 43 Rue Cuvier, 75005 Paris, France

Cell transformation leading to tumour development is a multistep process involving the activation of growth-stimulatory pathways (under the control of oncogenes) and the inactivation of growth-inhibitory pathways (under the control of tumour-suppressor genes). Inhibition of oncogenes and/or stimulation of tumour-suppressor genes represent new strategies that should lead i) to a better understanding of the different steps involved in tumourigenesis, and ii) to the development of new therapeutic approaches.

During the past years, oligonucleotide derivatives have been developed to selectively modulate gene expression. Several strategies can be contemplated [1] :
- in the *antisense* strategy, the oligonucleotide is targeted to a specific messenger RNA thereby inhibiting its translation into the corresponding protein [2] :
- an oligoribonucleotide can be engineered so as to induce cleavage of the target RNA (*ribozymes*) [3] ;
- in the *antigene* strategy, a double-stranded DNA sequence is the target of the oligonucleotide which is then expected to block transcription of the specific gene where the target is located [4].

Figure 1 gives a schematic representation of the different steps of gene expression where oligonucleotides can exert their biological effects. In addition, oligonucleotides can be used to trap proteins involved in gene expression [5]. Short double-stranded oligonucleotides bind transcription factors and thereby modulate gene transcription. This approach is expected to be less selective than the antisense or antigene strategies because transcription factors are usually involved in the control of several genes rather than a single one.

Here we will briefly review the basic principles underlying each strategy and then show how they have been applied to the inhibition of specific oncogenes in tumour cells.

Antisense RNAs and Ribozymes

Antisense RNAs are obtained by transcription of the sense strand of a gene or a fragment of a gene [6]. This requires the construction of an expression vector in which a gene fragment is placed under the control of a promoter in the reverse orientation as compared to the original gene. Upon transient transfection or after stable integration of the antisense construct, the antisense RNA that is synthesised hybridises with the corresponding messenger RNA to which it is fully complementary. Inhibition of mRNA translation is then expected to occur.

Regulatory RNAs are used by bacteria to control plasmid copy number or to modulate gene expression. In some cases the regulatory RNA arises from transcription of a regulatory gene that gives only partial complementarity to the controlled mRNA. The role of natural antisense RNAs in eukaryotes is still unclear [6]. Antisense RNAs can be considered as potential tools in gene therapy approaches rather than in chemotherapy.

Ribozymes [3] are short RNAs that are composed of 3 parts: 2 antisense sequences which are complementary to 2 sequences that flank the cleavage site, and a conserved sequence that allows the ribozyme-RNA

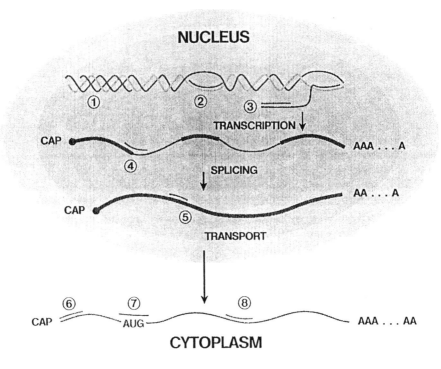

NUCLEUS

TRANSCRIPTION

CAP ● AAA . . . A

SPLICING

CAP ● AA . . . A

TRANSPORT

CAP ════════ AUG ──────────────── AAA . . . AA

CYTOPLASM

Fig. 1. Summary of the possible sites of sequence-specific action for oligonucleotides along the information flow from DNA to protein in a eukaryotic cell. Oligonucleotides could interfere: (i) with transcription by triple helix formation (1) on sequences containing contiguous purines (Pu) on one strand and pyrimidines (Py) on the other strand, by hybridisation to the locally opened loop created by RNA polymerase (2) or by hybridisation to nascent RNA (3); (ii) with splicing through hybridisation at intron-exon junctions (4); (iii) with the turn-over of spliced mRNA via, e.g., RNAse H-induced cleavage (5); (iv) with translation, through inhibition of the binding of initiation factors (6), inhibition of the assembly of ribosomal subunits at the start codon (7) or inhibition of polypeptide chain elongation (8) via RNase H-induced cleavage of the mRNA. Other processes such as capping and polyadenylation, interactions of snRNPs with pre-mRNAs in the splicing machinery, recruitment of stored mRNA into polysomes, nucleic acid-protein complexes are not illustrated in the Figure (adapted from reference 1).

complex to fold into the appropriate conformation so as to induce cleavage. The only sequence requirement on the target RNA is to possess a $5'GUN^{3'}$ sequence where N=U, C or A but not G and cleavage occurs on the 3'-side of N which is not paired to the antisense sequence of the ribozyme. Upon cleavage of the target RNA (messenger or viral), biological activity is lost. The cleavage reaction can be easily monitored *in vitro* but less so within cells due to further degradation of the cleaved products. In cells in culture it is difficult to distinguish the respective contributions of the ribozymic activity and the antisense effect that arises from binding of the ribozyme to its target sequence. Many studies are under way to improve the efficacy of ribozymes and to replace as many of the ribonucleotides as possible to make them resistant to nucleases [7-9].

An elegant example of the potential application of ribozymes to selective oncogene inactivation has been described [10]. Normal human Ha-*ras* mRNA has a GGU codon at position 12. Activation of this oncogene is due to point mutations in this codon. When GGU is converted to GUU (as in Ha-*ras* from a bladder carcinoma cell line called T24 or EJ), it becomes a target for a ribozyme which cleaves GUU after the second U but is unable to do so when the target contains the sequence GGU as in the normal mRNA.
Further experiments are clearly required to determine how ribozymes could be developed as drugs and delivered to tissues. In this respect the problems faced by ribozymes are similar to those raised by antisense or antigene oligonucleotides, except for the length (ribozymes have longer sequences) and the necessity of maintaining some *ribo*phospho-

diester linkages that will be sensitive to RNases.

Alternatively, a gene construct can be made to produce the ribozyme from within the cells. It remains to be seen whether ribozymes will have any advantage as compared to antisense RNAs. One clear difference will be the discrimination between 2 sequences arising from mutations (or translocation events) as exemplified above with the Ha-ras mRNA.

Antisense Oligonucleotides

Antisense Mechanisms

To recognise a specific sequence on a messenger RNA an oligonucleotide with a complementary sequence can be synthesised. The recognition involves Watson-Crick hydrogen bonding interactions between complementary bases. The first synthetic molecules used as antisense agents were oligodeoxyribonucleotides (oligo(dN)) because their chemical synthesis was (and still is) much easier than that of their ribo analogues.

The original idea behind the antisense strategy was that upon binding to a complementary sequence on a mRNA the oligonucleotide would inhibit translation of the mRNA by ribosomes. However, it became clear in the mid 80s that an oligonucleotide bound to the coding sequence of a mRNA would not be able to stop the translation machinery once it is launched on the mRNA. There are - at least - 2 mechanisms by which oligodeoxynucleotides inhibit mRNA translation :

- the oligo(dN)-mRNA hybrid is a substrate for an endogenous ribonuclease, called RNase H, which recognises DNA-RNA hybrids and cleaves exclusively the RNA part;
- an oligo(dN) bound to the 5'-untranslated region of a mRNA can inhibit binding or sliding of the 40S ribosomal subunit and/or the association of protein factors involved in translation initiation.

The first mechanism is probably an obligatory pathway for the antisense effect when the oligo(dN) is targeted to the coding sequence of the mRNA. The second mechanism is superimposed on the first when the oligo(dN) is targeted to the 5'-untranslated region of the mRNA.

Specificity of the Antisense Effect

An antisense oligonucleotide should be designed to recognise a single mRNA species within the mRNA population of a human cell. It has been calculated [11] that its minimum length should be between 11 and 15, depending on its base composition: 11 if it contains only Gs and Cs, 15 if it contains As and Ts (this difference accounts for the higher A.T. (60%) than G.C. (40%) content in human DNA). These numbers were calculated with the assumption that DNA base pairs are randomly distributed in the 4×10^9 bp-long human genome and that about 0.5% of this genome is transcribed as mRNA in a given cell type at a given time.

Antisense oligonucleotides should be chosen as short as possible to achieve a higher specificity under physiological conditions. This arises because the effect of mismatches on the binding energy decreases when the oligonucleotide length increases. Therefore, under physiological conditions (37°C, ionic conditions prevailing inside cell compartments), a shorter oligonucleotide should yield a higher discrimination between its complementary sequence and a sequence with a single base change. Of course, the oligonucleotide should have a minimum length i) to avoid its binding to fully complementary sequences that would otherwise be found in several mRNA species and ii) to achieve a strong enough binding under physiological conditions in order to have an inhibitory effect on the biological function (translation). Antisense oligonucleotides which have been shown to induce specific biological responses have usually been chosen in the range of 12 to 20 nucleotides. Shorter oligonucleotides can be used provided their hybrids with mRNAs are stabilised, e.g., by covalent attachment of an intercalating agent (see modified oligonucleotides, below).

Oligonucleotide Modifications

Oligonucleotides have been chemically modified to increase their nuclease resistance and their uptake by cells in culture. Oligophosphorothioates and dithioates still induce RNase H cleavage of an RNA target as do natural phosphodiester backbones. Oligophosphorothioates have been used to inhibit gene expression in several *in vitro* systems and in cell cultures [12]. They have been shown to inhibit HIV development. However, there is a non sequence-specific effect of these oligophosphorothioates on acute infection which might be due to their binding to the cell surface receptor CD4 and viral proteins such as reverse transcriptase and gp120 [13]. In contrast, a sequence-specific inhibition is observed in chronically-infected cells or if the oligophosphorothioates are added some time after cell infection.

Oligomethylphosphonates which are neutral derivatives (no negative charge on the phosphates) do not sustain RNase H activity on their target mRNA. They are expected to be active only when targeted to non-coding sequences. An oligomethylphosphonate complementary to an exon-intron junction was shown to inhibit splicing of immediate-early genes of Herpes Simplex Virus (HSV1) [14].

In oligo-[α]-deoxynucleotides the natural [ß]-anomers of nucleoside units have been changed to their synthetic [α]-anomers where the base is located on the same side as the 3'-OH with respect to the main sugar plane (as opposed to the 5'-OH in the [ß]-anomers). Oligo-[α]-deoxynucleotides are resistant to nucleases [15] but do not induce RNase H-mediated cleavage of their RNA substrate. Consequently, they are devoid of any antisense activity when targeted to coding sequences but may inhibit translation according to an RNase H-independent mechanism when targeted to the 5'-untranslated region [16-18].

Since RNase H has a strict requirement for ß-deoxyribo derivatives with phosphodiester or phosphorothioate backbones, it was of interest to determine whether mixed oligonucleotides would still induce RNase H cleavage. RNase H requires only 4-5 base pairs to achieve cleavage of the RNA part of an RNA-DNA hybrid. Oligonucleotides containing nuclease-resistant backbones (phosphoramidites) at both the 5'- and 3'-ends and 4-5 phosphodiesters in the centre are still active at inducing RNase H-mediated cleavage of

their RNA substrate while being highly resistant to exonucleases [19].

Other modifications have been introduced into oligonucleotides to improve their antisense efficacy. We early introduced intercalating agents as terminal substituents to increase the stability of oligonucleotide-mRNA complexes [20]. At the same time 3'-substitution of the oligonucleotide provided a protection against 3' --> 5' exonucleases which are the most active nucleases in plasma and inside cells. In addition, the intercalating agent enhanced cell uptake. All these properties make oligonucleotide-intercalator conjugates interesting substances to inhibit mRNA translation. They have been shown to prevent the cytopathic effect of influenza virus [21] and Simian Virus 40 [22] on cells in culture. Trypanosomes, the parasites responsible for spleeping sickness, were killed by an oligonucleotide-intercalator conjugate targeted to the common sequence which is present at the 5'-end of all trypanosomal mRNAs [23].

Oligonucleotides can be substituted by hydrophobic groups such as cholesterol [24,25]. These derivatives bind to lipoproteins: this binding increases their lifetime in plasma and opens the possibility that their cellular uptake occurs via LDL receptors [26].

Oligonucleotides can also be attached to reagents that can induce irreversible reactions in their target sequence [1,27,28]. Upon binding to a complementary sequence the reagent can be activated either chemically or photochemically to induce reactions such as cleavage of the target sequence or cross-linking of the 2 nucleic acids. A discussion of these different types of reactions is beyond the scope of this review; the reader is referred to recent reviews on the subject [1,27,28].

Oncogenes as Targets for Antisense Oligonucleotides

Oncogenes can be selected as targets for antisense oligonucleotides. If translation of an oncogene mRNA is blocked then one should expect to alter cell behaviour depending on whether the oncogene is involved in cell immortalisation or in cell transformation.

Discrimination Between Proto-Oncogene and Activated Oncogene

There are several situations where the activated oncogene can be selectively inhibited without any effect (or with weaker effects) on the corresponding proto-oncogene

- when activation results from a point mutation. This has been documented in the case of the Ha-*ras* oncogene from T24 cells (a bladder carcinoma cell line) where Ha-*ras* is activated by a point mutation on codon 12 [29]. An antisense oligonucleotide targeted to the mutated sequence induced RNAse H cleavage of the mutated mRNA whereas a much weaker effect was seen on the normal mRNAs. An inhibition of T24 cell proliferation was demonstrated. The discrimination between the mutated and normal sequence is due to the destabilisation of the oligonucleotide-mRNA hybrid resulting from a mismatch at the point mutation site. Alternatively, a ribozyme can be used to discriminate a mutant from the normal Ha-*ras* mRNA [10];
- when activation results from translocation creating a new fusion gene. This occurs, for instance, in chronic myelogenous leukaemia (CML) where a *bcr-abl* hybrid gene arising from a translocation between chromosomes 9 and 22 is responsible for cell transformation [30]; in acute promyelocytic leukaemia (APL) where a t (15;17) translocation fuses the retinoic acid receptor α (RARα) gene to *myl* gene resulting in the synthesis of a *myl*/RARα fusion mRNA [31]; in B-cell lymphomas where a t (14;18) translation generates chimeric mRNAs involving a *bcl2*-immunoglobulin fusion [32]. An antisense oligonucleotide targeted to the chimeric *bcr-abl* junction was shown to selectively suppress growth of leukaemia cells from CML blast crisis patients without any effect on normal progenitor cells [33];
- when transcription is initiated from an aberrant promoter without translocation. In many Burkitt lymphomas c-*myc* transcription starts in the first intron of the normal gene. Consequently, the mRNA contains sequences which are not found in the normal c-*myc* mRNA. It was recently shown that a 21-mer antisense oligonucleotide directed against the intron sequence was able to inhibit proliferation of tumour cells

that expressed the abnormal transcript but not in cells containing the normal transcript [34];
- when alternative splicing or deletion mutations create a new mRNA species containing sequences which are not found in the original mRNA. This occurs, for example, in some gliomas where the EGF-receptor mRNA arises from an in-frame deletion mutation [35]. There is no report yet on antisense application to these tumour cells.

Inhibition of Oncogene Expression

An antisense oligonucleotide targeted to an oncogene mRNA can be expected to have selective effects on tumour cell proliferation even when the target is also present in normal cells. This occurs in many cases of cell transformation where abnormal expression of the proto-oncogene is sufficient to deregulate cell growth as a result of, for instance, gene amplification or enhanced transcription (or translation).

The *myc* oncogenes have received a great deal of attention. The human promyelocytic cell line HL 60 has been used as a model because it overexpresses c-*myc* as a result of gene amplification and can be induced to differentiate into either monocytes or granulocytes by various agents. This differentiation is associated with a decrease in c-*myc* protein synthesis. A 15-mer antisense oligonucleotide targeted to the first 5 codons of the c-*myc* mRNA was shown to induce a sequence-specific reduction in c-*myc* expression which was accompanied by inhibition of cell proliferation and by granulocytic differentiation [36,37]. By "walking" along the human c-*myc* mRNA with 15-mer oligonucleotides the highest antisense efficacy was obtained when the target was the 5'-cap untranslated region [38]. The N-*myc* oncogene was also inhibited by a 15-mer antisense oligonucleotide targeted to the translation initiation site in a neuroepithelioma cell line [39]. The results provided a clear example of the sequence selectivity of the antisense effect because the closely related c-*myc* gene was not affected by the anti-N-*myc* oligonucleotide.

The role of the c-*myb* gene in a number of cells has been addressed by using antisense oligonucleotides to reduce c-*myb* protein expression (T-cell leukaemias, normal T-cells and bone marrow progenitors, myeloid leukaemia). An 18-mer oligonucleotide targeted to codons 2-7 was shown to inhibit proliferation of myeloid leukaemia cell lines [40] as well as DNA synthesis in T-leukaemia cells. Normal and leukaemic haematopoietic cells manifest differential sensitivity to inhibitory effects of c-*myb* antisense oligodeoxynucleotides [41], suggesting that such oligonucleotides could be used as *ex vivo* bone marrow purging agents.

The *ras* family of oncogenes has been investigated as a potential target for antisense oligonucleotides. In the experiments reported in the preceding paragraph it was shown that an antisense oligonucleotide or a ribozyme directed towards a region comprising the mutation could discriminate between the proto-oncogene and the oncogene [10,29]. All 3 *ras* genes (Ha-*ras*, Ki-*ras*, N-*ras*) are activated by point mutations and therefore are amenable to the same strategy. *Ras* mRNA sequences that are outside the point mutation have also been used as targets for antisense oligonucleotides. The 5'-cap untranslated region of the Ha-*ras* gene appears to be the most efficient target for maximum inhibition of p21 synthesis [42]. The targets are identical in both the normal and the mutated genes when the oligonucleotide does not overlap the mutation; therefore, no discrimination is expected between the proto-oncogene and the oncogene.

Cellular receptors, cytokines, growth factors etc. can be chosen as targets for antisense oligonucleotides aimed at inhibiting cell proliferation. This has been particularly well demonstrated when autocrine growth loops are involved. Both colony stimulating factor CSF-1 [43] and its receptor encoded by the c-*fms* gene [44] can be inhibited by antisense oligonucleotides resulting in inhibition of proliferation of autocrine cells [43] or differentiation of HL 60 cells induced by phorbol esters [44]. Certain human myeloma cell lines are characterised by an IL-6 autocrine growth loop which can be blocked by an anti-IL 6 oligonucleotide [45]. The growth of IL-2-and IL-4 dependent cell lines can also be selectively inhibited by antisense oligonucleotides [46]. Antisense oligonucleotides targeted to basic fibroblast growth factor (bFGF) inhibit

malignant melanoma cell proliferation and colony formation in soft agar [47].

The Anti-Gene Strategy

In the antisense approach the oligonucleotide is targeted to a messenger RNA and is thus expected to inhibit translation. Viral RNAs can also be used as targets for complementary oligonucleotides that will inhibit either replication or viral gene expression [13,48]. More recently it has become clear that DNA itself could be the target for oligonucleotides that would inhibit the first step of gene expression, namely, transcription [49,50]. We have called this new approach the "anti-gene" strategy [1,4]. The molecular basis for the recognition of a DNA double helical sequence by an oligonucleotide is summarised in Figure 2. Thymine and protonated cytosine can form 2 hydrogen bonds with A.T and G.C Watson-Crick base pairs, respectively, generating base-triplets T.AxT and C.GxC+ where the dot indicates Watson-Crick hydrogen bonding in the base pairs T.A and C.G and the cross refers to the so-called Hoogsteen hydrogen bonds illustrated in Figure 2. Therefore, an oligonucleotide containing T and C can recognise a homopurine.homopyrimidine sequence on duplex DNA and form a local triple helix. It binds to the major groove of DNA in a parallel orientation with respect to the homopurine sequence. Oligonucleotides containing G and T or G and A nucleotides can also bind to homopurine.homopyrimidine sequences of DNA [51,52]. Although the base triplets C.GxG and T.AxT or T.AxA are not isomorphous (whereas T.AxT and C.GxC+ are isomorphous), G/T and G/A oligonucleotides may form more stable triple helices under physiological conditions because they do not require base protonation. In contrast, cytosine protonation (favoured by low pH) is required to form the C.G x C+ base triplet. Replacement of cytosine by 5-methylcytosine allows more stable complexes to be formed at neutral pH.

In order to recognise a single sequence on double helical DNA in human cells, a triple helix-forming oligonucleotide must have a minimum length of about 17 bases [11]. Triple

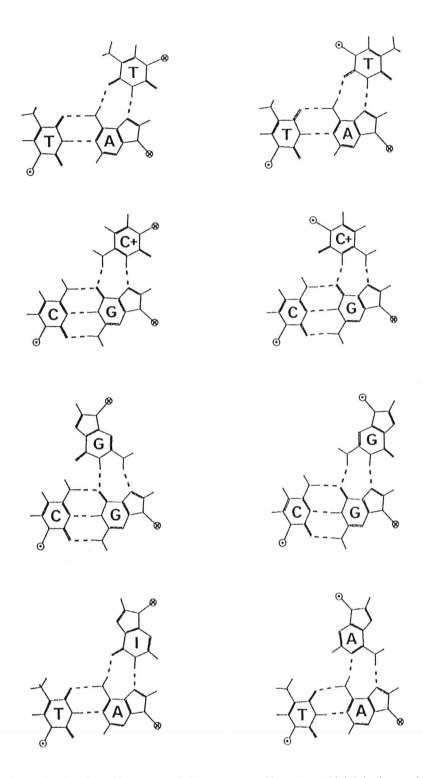

Fig. 2. Triple helix formation involves Hoogsteen (left) or reverse Hoogsteen (right) hydrogen bonding of bases to Watson-Crick T.A. or C.G. base pairs. C$^+$ indicates protonated cytosine.

helix formation by oligonucleotides is strongly stabilised when oligonucleotides are covalently linked to intercalating agents [53] (Fig. 3). Triple-strand forming oligonucleotides can also be equipped with substituents that can induce irreversible reactions in their target sequence such as cross-linking of the oligonucleotide or cleavage of the DNA

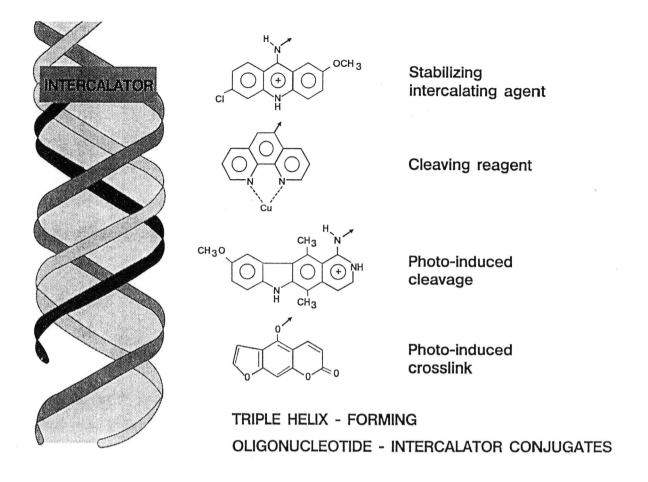

Stabilizing
intercalating agent

Cleaving reagent

Photo-induced
cleavage

Photo-induced
crosslink

TRIPLE HELIX - FORMING

OLIGONUCLEOTIDE - INTERCALATOR CONJUGATES

Fig. 3. Oligonucleotide targeting to double-stranded DNA. A homopyrimidine oligonucleotide (black ribbon) can bind to the major groove of double helical DNA at a homopurine.homopyrimidine sequence. The oligonucleotide can be substituted by an intercalating agent that stabilises the triplex or induces irreversible reactions in the target as indicated in the right part of the Figure.

strands [49,50,54,55]. Recently we have shown that the 2 strands of DNA can be cross-linked by a psoralen-oligonucleotide conjugate under UV-irradiation at the specific sequence where the oligonucleotide forms a triple helix [56] (see Fig. 3).
Oligonucleotide-directed triple helix formation inhibits association of sequence-specific DNA binding proteins such as restriction enzymes or transcription factors [51,57-59]. It is thus expected that triple helices will interfere with biological processes such as transcription and replication. A triple helix-forming oligonucleotide does block transcription of the c-*myc* gene because it inhibits binding of a transcription factor to one of the regulatory sequences upstream of the transcription start site [51]. More recently, oligonucleotide-directed triple helix formation was shown to in-

hibit the synthesis of the mRNA of IL2 receptor subunit α in cultured cells [60]. Replication of Simian Virus SV40 DNA was reported to be inhibited in CV1 cells treated with an oligonucleotide-intercalator conjugate [22]. In all cases it remains to be demonstrated that the effects observed on cells in culture are due to triple helix formation and not to binding of the oligonucleotide to other targets. A direct proof of triple helix formation *in vivo* might use oligonucleotides carrying reactive groups that can be activated to induce an irreversible reaction (e.g., cross-linking) at the specific site on DNA where the oligonucleotide is bound.
As discussed above in the case of the antisense strategy, triple helix-forming oligonucleotides can be modified to make them resistant to nucleases. We have shown that oligo-[α]-deoxynucleotides can bind to the DNA

double helix at homopurine.homopyrimidine sequences [49,61,62]. Substitution of the [α]-anomers of nucleotide units to the natural [ß]-anomers make these oligonucleotides highly resistant to nucleases [15].

The development of triple helix-forming oligonucleotides as potential tools to control gene expression at the transcriptional level is still in its infancy. The only published application dealing with oncogene inhibition used the c-*myc* oncogene as a target *in vitro* [51] and in cell cultures [63]. The forthcoming years will certainly see a burst in publications dealing with the anti-gene strategy applied to specific cellular genes, including oncogenes, as was observed in the mid 80s with the antisense strategy.

Further Developments

The problems faced by anti-gene oligonucleotides as far as potential therapeutic applications are concerned are similar to those raised by anti-sense oligonucleotides. Both cell uptake and intracellular distribution ought to be improved to increase the efficacy of oligonucleotides. In the antisense strategy the target is either the mRNA in the cytosol or the pre-mRNA in the nucleus; in the anti-gene strategy the DNA target is located in the nucleus. Oligonucleotides appear to be taken up by endocytosis and therefore a large part of the oligonucleotide might be trapped in endocytic vesicles within the cytoplasm [64]. Recent experiments have shown that upon microinjection in cells oligonucleotides are rapidly concentrated in the nucleus [65]. Therefore, the mode of oligonucleotide delivery is expected to play an important role in determining the efficacy of their biological effects. There are many steps dealing with pharmacokinetics, tissue distribution, bioavailability, delivery systems etc. which are being addressed by several laboratories [66]. Toxicological problems have not been addressed yet, except for acute toxicity studies in mice and rats [13,64]. When dealing with modified oligonucleotides degradation products might exhibit toxic effects. In addition, side effects arising from binding of oligonucleotides to targets other than nucleic acids, e.g., proteins, must be carefully examined.

The results presently available provide a rational basis for the development of highly selective therapeutic approaches. Tumour-specific targets can be identified but it remains to be demonstrated whether inhibition of expression of these target genes can be achieved *in vivo* and whether this approach can be qualified as useful cancer chemotherapy.

REFERENCES

1   Hélène C and Toulmé JJ: Specific regulation of gene expression by antisense, sense and antigene nucleic acids. Biochimica et Biophysica Acta 1990 (1049):99-125
2   Hélène C: Rational design of sequence-specific gene inhibitors based on antisense and antigene oligonucleotides. Eur J Cancer 1991 (27):1466-1471
3   Rossi JJ and Sarver N: RNA enzymes (ribozymes) as antiviral therapeutic agents. Trends in Biotechnology 1990 (8):179-183
4   Hélène C: The anti-gene strategy: control of gene expression by triplex-forming-oligonucleotides. Anti-Cancer Drug Design 1991: December issue
5   Bielinska A, Shivdasani RA, Zhang L and Nabel GJ: Regulation of gene expression with double-stranded phosphorothioate oligonucleotides. Science 1990 (250):997-1000
6   Takayama KM and Inouye M: Antisense RNA. Critical Reviews in Biochemistry and Molecular Biology 1990 (25):155-184
7   Herschlag D: Implications of ribozyme kinetics for targeting the cleavage of specific RNA molecules in vivo: more isn't always better. Proc Natl Acad Sci USA 1991 (88):6921-6925
8   Smith JB and Dinter-Gottlieb G: Antigenomic Hepatitis delta virus ribozymes self-cleave in 18 M formamide. Nucleic Acids Res 1991 (19):1285-1289
9   Pieken WA, Olsen DB, Benseler F, Aurup H and Eckstein F: Kinetic characterization of ribonuclease-resistant 2'-modified hammerhead ribozymes. Science 1991 (253):314-317
10 Koizumi M, Hayase Y, Iwai S, Kamiya H, Inouye H and Ohtsuka E: Design of RNA enzymes distinguishing a single base mutation in RNA. Nucleic Acids Res 1989 (17):7059-7071
11 Hélène C and Toulmé JJ: Control of gene expression by oligodeoxynucleotides covalently linked to intercalating agents and nucleic acid-cleaving reagents. In: Cohen JS (ed) Oligodeoxynucleotides: Antisense Inhibitors of Gene Expression. MacMillan Press, London 1989 pp 137-172
12 Stein CA and Cohen JS: Phosphorothioate oligodeoxynucleotide analogues. In: Cohen JS (ed) Oligodeoxynucleotides: Antisense Inhibitors of Gene Expression. MacMillan Press, London 1989 pp 97-117
13 Agrawal S and Sarin PS: Antisense oligonucleotides: gene regulation and chemotherapy of AIDS. Advanced Drug Delivery Reviews 1991 (6):251-270
14 Kulka M, Smith CC, Aurelian L, Fishelevich R, Meade K, Miller P and Ts'o POP: Site specificity of the inhibitory effects of oligo(nucleoside methylphosphonate)s complementary to the acceptor splice junction of herpes simplex virus type 1 immediate early mRNA 4. Proc Natl Acad Sci USA 1989 (86):6868-6872
15 Cazenave C, Chevrier M, Thuong NT, and Hélène C: Rate of degradation of [α]- and [ß]-oligodeoxy-nucleotides in Xenopus oocytes. Implications for anti-messenger strategies. Nucleic Acids Res 1987 (15):10507-10521
16 Cazenave C, Stein CA, Loreau N, Thuong NT, Neckers LM, Subasinghe C, Hélène C, Cohen JS and Toulmé JJ: Comparative inhibition of rabbit globin mRNA translation by modified antisense oligodeoxynucleotides. Nucleic Acids Res 1989 (17):4255-4273
17 Bertrand JR, Imbach JL, Paoletti C and Malvy C: Comparative activity of α- and ß-anomeric oligonucleotides on rabbit ß-globin synthesis: inhibitory effect of cap targeted α-oligonucleotides. Biochem Biophys Res Commun 1989 (164):311-318
18 Boiziau C, Kurfurst R, Cazenave C, Roig V, Thuong NT and Toulmé JJ: Inhibition of translation initiation by antisense oligonucleotides via an RNase-H independent mechanism. Nucleic Acids Res 1991 (19):1113-1119
19 Dagle JM, Andracki ME, Devine RJ and Walder JA: Physical properties of oligonucleotides containing phosphoramidate-modified internucleoside linkages. Nucleic Acids Res 1991 (19):1805-1810
20 Asseline U, Thuong NT and Hélène C: New substances with high and specific affinity toward nucleic acid sequences: intercalating agents covalently linked to an oliodeoxynucleotide. CR Acad Sci Paris 1983 (297): 369-372
21 Zérial A, Thuong NT and Hélène C: Selective inhibition of the cytopathic effect of type A influenza viruses by oligodeoxynucleotides covalently linked to an intercalating agent. Nucleic Acids Res 1987 (15):9909-9919
22 Birg F, Praseuth D, Zérial A, Thuong NT, Asseline U, Le Doan T and Hélène C: Inhibition of simian virus 40 DNA replication in CV-1 cells by an oligodeoxynucleotide covalently linked to an intercalating agent. Nucleic Acids Res 1990 (18):2901-2908
23 Verspieren P, Cornelissen AWCA, Thuong NT, Hélène C and Toulmé JJ: An acridine-linked oligodeoxynucleotide targeted to the common 5' end of trypanosome mRNAs kills cultured parasites. Gene 1987 (61):307-315
24 Boutorin AS, Gus'Kova LV, Ivanova EM, Kobetz ND, Zarytova VF, Ryte AS, Yurchenko LV and Vlassov VV: Synthesis of alkylating oligonucleotide derivatives containing cholesterol or phenazinium residues at their 3'-terminus and their interaction with DNA within mammalian cells. FEBS Letters 1989 (254):129-132
25 Letsinger RL, Zhang G, Sun DK, Ikeuchi T and Sarin PS: Cholesterol-conjugated oligonucleotides: synthesis, properties, and activity as inhibitors of replication of human immunodeficiency virus in cell culture. Proc Natl Acad Sci USA 1989 (86):6553-6556
26 De Smidt C, Le Doan T, De Falco S and Van Berkel T: Association of antisense oligonucleotides with lipoproteins prolongs the plasma half life and modifies the tissue distribution. Nucleic Acids Res 1991 (19):4695-4700
27 Knorre DG, Vlassov VV, Zarytova VF: Oligonucleotides linked to reactive groups. In: Cohen JS (ed) Oligodeoxynucleotides: Antisense Inhibitors of Gene Expression. MacMillan Press, London 1989 pp 173-210

28 Hélène C, Le Doan T and Thuong NT: Sequence targeted photochemical reactions in single-stranded and double-stranded nucleic acids by oligonucleotide-photosensitizer conjugates. In: Nielsen PE (ed) Photochemical Probes in Biochemistry. Kluwer Academic Publishers 1989 pp 219-299

29 Saison-Behmoaras T, Tocqué B, Rey I, Chassignol M, Thuong NT and Hélène C: Short modified antisense oligonucleotides directed against Ha-ras point mutation induce selective cleavage of the mRNA and inhibit T24 cells proliferation. EMBO J 1991 (10):1111-1118

30 Champlin RE and Golde DW: Chronic myelogenous leukemia: recent advances. Blood 1985 (65):1039-1047

31 De Thé H, Chomienne C, Lanotte M, Degos L and Dejean A: The t(15;17) translocation of acute promyelocytic leukaemia fuses the retinoic acid receptor α gene to a novel transcribed locus. Nature 1990 (347) 558-561

32 Seto M, Jaeger U, Hockett RD, Graninger W, Bennett S, Goldman P and Korsmeyer SJ: Alternative promoters and exons, somatic mutation and deregulation of the Bcl-2-Ig fusion gene in lymphoma. EMBO J 1988 (7):123-131

33 Szczylik C, Skorsky T, Nicolaides NC, Manzella L, Malaguarnera L, Venturelli D, Gewirtz AM and Calabretta B: Selective inhibition of leukemia cell proliferation by BCR-ABL antisense oligodeoxynucleotides. Science 1991 (253):562-565

34 McManaway ME, Neckers LM, Loke SL, Al-Nasser AA, Redner RL, Shiramizu BT, Goldschmidts WL, Huber BE, Bhatia K and Magrath IT: Tumour-specific inhibition of lymphoma growth by an antisense oligodeoxynucleotide. Lancet 1990 (335):808-811

35 Humphrey PA, Wong AJ, Vogelstein B et al: Anti-synthetic peptide antibody reacting at the fusion junction of deletion-mutant epidermal growth factor receptors in human glioblastoma. Proc Natl Acad Sci USA 1990 (87):4207-4211

36 Wickstrom EL, Bacon TA, Gonzalez A, Lyman GH and Wickstrom E: Human promyelocytic leukemia HL-60 cell proliferation and c-myc protein expression are inhibited by an antisense pentadecadeoxynucleotide. Proc Natl Acad Sci USA 1988 (85):1028-1032

37 Holt JT, Redner RL and Nienhuis AW: An oligomer complementary to c-myc mRNA inhibits proliferation of HL-60 promyelocytic cells and induces differentiation. Mol Cell Biol 1988 (8):963-973

38 Bacon TA and Wickstrom E: Walking along human c-myc mRNA with antisense oligonucleotides: maximum efficacy at the 5' cap region. Oncogene Res 1991 (6):13-19

39 Rosolen A, Whitesell L, Ikegaki N, Kennett RH and Neckers LM: Antisense inhibition of single copy N-myc expression results in decreased cell growth without reduction of c-myc protein in a neuroepithelioma cell line. Cancer Res 1990 (50): 6316-6322

40 Anfossi G, Gewirtz AM and Calabretta B: An oligomer complementary to c-myb-encoded mRNA inhibits proliferation of human myeloid leukemia cell lines. Proc Natl Acad Sci USA 1989 (86):3379-3383

41 Calabretta B, Sims RB, Valtieri M, Caracciolo D, Szczylik C, Venturelli D, Ratajczak M, Beran M and Gewirtz AM: Normal and leukemic hematopoietic cells manifest differential sensitivity to inhibitory effects of c-myb antisense oligonucleotides: An in vitro study relevant to bone marrow purging. Proc Natl Acad Sci USA 1991 (88):2351-2355

42 Daaka Y and Wickstrom E: Target dependence of antisense oligodeoxynucleotide inhibition of c-Ha-ras p21 expression and focus formation in T24-transformed NIH3T3 cell. Oncogene Res 1990 (5):279-289

43 Birchenall RM, Ferrer C, Ferris D, Falk LA, Kasper J, White G and Ruscetti FW: Inhibition of murine monocyte proliferation by a colony-stimulating factor-1 antisense oligodeoxynucleotide. Evidence for autocrine regulation. J Immunol 1990 (145):3290-3296

44 Wu J, Zhu JQ, Han KK and Zhu DX: The role of the c-fms oncogene in the regulation of HL-60 cell differentiation. Oncogene 1990 (5):873-877

45 Schwab G, Siegall CB, Aarden LA, Neckers L and Nordan RP: Characterization of an interleukin-6-mediated autocrine growth loop in the human multiple myeloma cell line U266. Blood 1991 (77):587-593

46 Harel-Bellan A, Durum S, Muegge K, Abbas A and Farrar W: Specific inhibition of lymphokine biosynthesis and autocrine growth using antisense oligonucleotides in Th1 and Th2 helper T cell clones. J Exp Med 1988 (168):2309-2318

47 Becker D, Meier CB and Herlyn M: Proliferation of human malignant melanomas is inhibited by antisense oligonucleotides targeted against basic fibroblast growth factor. EMBO J 1989 (8):3685-3691

48 Zamecnik PC and Stephenson ML: Inhibition of Rous sarcoma virus replication and cell transformation by a specific oligodeoxynucleotide. Proc Natl Acad Sci USA 1978 (75):280-284

49 Le Doan T, Perrouault L, Praseuth D, Habhoub N, Decout JL, Thuong NT, Lhomme J and Hélène C: Sequence-specific recognition, photocrosslinking and cleavage of the DNA double helix by an oligo-a-thymidylate covalently linked to an azidoproflavine derivative. Nucleic Acids Res 1987 (15):7749-7760

50 Moser HE and Dervan PB: Sequence-specific cleavage of double helical DNA by triple helix formation. Science 1987 (238):645-650

51 Cooney M, Czernuszewicz G, Postel EH, Flint SJ and Hogan ME: Site-specific oligonucleotide binding represses transcription of the human c-myc gene in vitro. Science 1988 (241):456-459

52 Beal PA and Dervan PB: Second structural motif for recognition of DNA by oligonucleotide-directed triple-helix formation. Science 1991 (251):1360-1363

53 Sun JS, François JC, Montenay-Garestier T, Saison-Behmoaras T, Roig V, Thuong NT and Hélène C: Sequence-specific intercalating agents: intercalation at specific sequences on duplex DNA via major groove recognition by oligonucleotide-

intercalator conjugates. Proc Natl Acad Sci USA 1989 (86):9198-9202

54 François JC, Saison-Behmoaras T, Barbier C, Chassignol M, Thuong NT and Hélène C: Sequence-specific recognition and cleavage of duplex DNA via triple-helix formation by oligonucleotides covalently linked to a phenanthroine-copper chelate. Proc Natl Acad Sci USA 1989 (86):9702-9706

55 Fedorova OS, Knorre DG, Podust LM and Zaritova VF: Complementary addressed modification of double-stranded DNA within a ternary complex. FEBS Letters 1988 (228):273-276

56 Takasugi M, Guendouz A, Chassignol M, Decout JL, Lhomme J, Thuong NT and Hélène C: Sequence-specific photo-induced cross-linking of the two strands of double-helical DNA by a psoralen covalently linked to a triple helix-forming oligonucleotide. Proc Natl Acad Sci USA 1991 (88):5602-5606

57 Maher LJ, Wold B and Dervan PB: Inhibition of DNA binding proteins by oligonucleotide-directed triple helix formation. Science 1989 (245):725-730

58 François JC, Saison-Behmoaras T, Thuong NT, Hélène C: Inhibition of restriction endonuclease cleavage via triple helix formation by homopyrimidine oligonucleotides. Biochemistry 1989 (28):9617-9619

59 Hanvey JC, Shimizu M and Wells RD: Site-specific inhibition of EcoRI restriction/modification enzymes by a DNA triple helix. Nucleic Acids Res 1990 (18):157-161

60 Orson FM, Thomas DW, McShan WM, Kessler DJ and Hogan ME: Oligonucleotide inhibition of IL2Rα mRNA transcription by promoter region collinear triplex formation in lymphocytes. Nucleic Acids Res 1991 (19):3435-3441

61 Praseuth D, Perrouault L, Le Doan T, Chassignol M, Thuong NT and Hélène C: Sequence-specific binding and photocrosslinking of α and ß oligodeoxynucleotides to the major groove of DNA via triple-helix formation. Proc Natl Acad Sci USA 1988 (85):1349-1353

62 Sun JS, Giovannangeli C, François JC, Kurfurst R, Montenay-Garestier T, Asseline U, Saison-Behmoaras T, Thuong NT and Hélène C: Triple-helix formation by α-oligodeoxynucleotides and α-oligodeoxynucleotide-intercalator conjugates. Proc Natl Acad Sci USA 1991 (88):6023-6027

63 Postel EH, Flint SJ, Kessler DJ and Hogan ME: Evidence that a triplex-forming oligodeoxyribonucleotide binds to the c-myc promoter in HeLa cells, thereby reducing c-myc mRNA levels. Proc Natl Acad Sci USA 1991 (88):8227-8231

64 Jaroszewski JW and Cohen JS: Cellular uptake of antisense oligodeoxynucleotides. Advanced Drug Delivery Reviews 1991 (6):235-250

65 Leonetti JP, Mechti N, Degols G, Gagnor C and Lebleu B: Intracellular distribution of microinjected antisense oligonucleotides. Proc Natl Acad Sci USA 1991 (88):2702-2706

66 Zon G: Oligonucleotide analogues as potential chemotherapeutic agents. Pharmaceutical Res 1988 (5):539-549

Prospects for Biological and Gene Therapies

Karol Sikora and Andres Guiterrez

Department of Clinical Oncology, Royal Postgraduate Medical School, Hammersmith Hospital, Du Cane Road, London W12 ONN, United Kingdom

We now know that cancer is a disorder of somatic cell genetics resulting in a clone of cells with an abnormal pattern of growth control. Conventional cancer therapy aims to bring about the selective destruction of the tumour, leaving as much as possible of normal tissue intact. The fundamental stumbling block of surgery and radiotherapy is the problem of tumour invasion and spread outside areas directly accessible to these modalities of treatment. The problem with chemotherapy is its low therapeutic ratio for many tumours and the fact that drug resistance may rapidly supervene or be present from the outset. Despite the encouraging success of chemotherapy for a variety of rare tumour types, in the vast majority of human solid cancers such treatment has had little impact on survival. This is disappointing considering the tremendous efforts of the last 20 years.

Biological approaches to the treatment of cancer began with the realisation that under certain circumstances there may be not only recognition of tumour cells by the host immune response but also an effective destructive mechanism. Whilst clear-cut evidence for the immunogenicity of tumours can be obtained from a variety of rodent model systems, evidence for an effective immune mechanism against the majority of human tumours is elusive. The last decade has seen the use of modern molecular biology to isolate genes and subsequently produce in pharmaceutical quantities a range of cytokines, many of which are involved in the control of the immune system. Some of these, such as the interferons and interleukins, have already been demonstrated to have limited efficacy against specific human tumours [1], although their mechanism of action is unclear [2].

Against the background of relative stagnation in terms of cancer therapy, we have seen remarkable developments in our understanding of the molecular basis of growth control. Oncogenes and tumour suppressor genes are clearly part of the normal human genome - vital in the transduction of physiological signals from the outside of the cell to its nucleus [3]. Subversion of this apparatus by a variety of mechanisms can cause cancer. At the moment the picture is confusing. The precise molecular pathogenesis of even a single type of cancer is not yet understood. Almost certainly a series of events is necessary for a tumour to emerge. As we go through this decade it is likely that the majority of the human genome will be sequenced, allowing a comparison between cells exhibiting abnormal growth patterns and their normal counterparts. Furthermore, the transcriptional control of several genes will be elucidated in detail and an understanding of tissue differentiation will emerge. This in turn will explain how different blocks of genes are expressed under different circumstances.

We are already beginning to see prognostic predictions by the use of genetic analysis in breast cancer, (amplification of *erb* B2), neuroblastoma (N-*myc* amplification) and *ras* mutations (adenocarcinoma of the lung) [4]. Further prognostic predictions will almost certainly uncover targets for future therapy. At a purely technical level, gene manipulation is becoming easier. Homologous recombination, retroviral shuttle vectors and antisense technology together with the power of the analytical tools, such as the polymerase chain reaction, will revolutionise our ability to manipulate cells in culture and perhaps whole organisms. Several clinical protocols

Table 1. Recombinant DNA Advisory Committee (NIH, Washington) cancer approvals

Gene	Cell	Investigator	Date
neo R	TIL	Rosenberg	January 89
TNF	TIL	Rosenberg	June 90
TK	ca	Freeman	July 91
IL-2	ca	Rosenberg	July 91
MHC	ca	Nabel	-

for human gene therapy have been given approval by the Recombinant DNA Advisory Committee (RAC) of National Institute of Health, Washington (Table 1). In each case, the goal of these protocols is the enhancement of the anti-tumour immune response in the host. Nevertheless, the potential of gene transfer in cancer goes beyond improving the efficiency of the immune system against the malignant cell. It could well result in novel approaches to halt the malignant behaviour of tumour cells directly.

This review will consider the prospects for biological and interventional gene therapy as methods for selectively destroying tumour cells in patients.

Gene Therapy

Principles

Gene therapy can be divided into two types, somatic and germ cell. The former refers to the insertion of a normal exogenous gene into somatic cells in order to correct an abnormality or deficiency of a specific protein. Somatic gene therapy can be carried out by transfecting the new gene in the presence of the old abnormal gene (addition therapy) or by attempting to specifically replace a defective gene by inserting a new one at the same site, using homologous recombination. In neither case will the genetic information be passed on to future generations. This is the type of technology that is required for the treatment of cancer. Germ cell transfection poses considerable ethical dilemmas and has little role to play in cancer therapy. It is possible that at some point in the future it

could be used to develop preventive strategies for the disease.

The diploid human genome consists of 6 x 10^9 base pairs (bp). A single chromosome contains a 120 x 10^6 (bp). Most genes are 20 x 10^3 bp in length. Considerable effort is currently going into the development of somatic gene therapy for single gene disorders such as adenosine deaminase immunodeficiency and thalassaemia [5]. These diseases would seem to be more amenable to this approach than a complex polygenic disorder such as cancer. However, there are several systems that have been explored in malignancy to enhance the selective destruction of tumour versus normal cells.

Delivery Systems

Techniques to inject a functional new gene into a cell are critical for successful therapy. There are two main methods, physical and virus mediated. Physical methods include transfection by calcium phosphate precipitation, electroporation, micro-injection, protoplast fusion, liposomal transfer or receptor mediated delivery [6]. More recently, interesting studies using the direct injection of vectors containing the dystrophin gene into murine muscle have shown at least short-term expression of this protein in cells surrounding the injection site [7]. Viral transfer using eco or amphotrophic retroviruses have been the most widely used due to their efficiency of injection. Modified adenovirus and herpes simplex virus have also been investigated due to their ability to infect specific tissues such as epithelial cells [8].

A major hurdle to overcome in cancer is the need for *in vivo* transfer. A cell line *in vitro* can relatively easily be transfected, but a solid tumour less so. There have been a several attempts at *in vivo* transfection through various routes including intraperitoneal, intravenous, intra-arterial, intrahepatic, intramuscular and intratracheal injection, using both physical and viral methods [9].

Expression

Major efforts have gone into improving the expression of genes once they are inserted into their target cells. These have included the use of selective promoters to efficiently drive transcription of the transfected genes. A reporter gene system is normally used to trace the efficiency of the insertion [10]. This may allow for a selective process, so enhancing the success of transfer.

Two major problems remain important limitations in mammalian cell transfection. The first is a much lower efficiency of gene expression in comparison to prokaryotic systems, with considerable differences existing between various eukaryotic cell lines. In contrast to rodent cells for example, primate and human cells can only integrate a small amount of foreign DNA (approximately 6 Kb), so that only 10-30% of clones selected for the expression of one transcription unit will also contain a second unit in intact form [11]. The second problem is the short-lived response obtained after successful transfection (at the most a few months) regardless of the methods employed [12]. We know very little about the processing steps within the cell. Clearly, there are problems of degradation by extracellular nucleases, absorption onto the cells, uptake into the cells, transport from cytoplasm to nucleus, ligation to DNA, mutation, the expression of unintegrated DNA and finally transcription control of the transgene. The evolution of safe, controllable gene delivery and expression systems is vital for successful therapy

Biological Approaches to Cancer

Recombinant Drugs

Although drugs produced by recombinant DNA technology are not directly a form of gene therapy, they rely on exactly the same technology. This group now includes cytokines, growth factors, growth factor antagonists, humanised monoclonal antibodies, toxin-antibody immunoconjugates, toxin-ligand conjugates and single-chain antigen binding proteins. So far there has been limited usefulness of some of these agents in cancer. The development of selectively toxic molecules has proven difficult. Despite tremendous efforts to produce specific monoclonal antibodies with high tumour affinity,

the actual selectivity of even the best of these agents is relatively limited. This almost certainly explains the currently poor clinical results. However, improvements in molecular design and the identification of novel specific molecular targets may enhance this approval.

Informational Drugs

Informational drugs can be defined as synthesised molecules that carry biological information which allows them to act in a specific manner. Oligonucleotides, ribozymes and specific proteases act at different but specific levels of the transcription system. These compounds can be of low molecular weight and therefore have considerable potential to reach tumour cell targets in vivo. Major problems include cell permeability, chemical stability, targeting, scale up and toxicity [13].

Antisense oligodeoxynucleotides are small synthetic nucleotide sequences formulated to be complementary to specific DNA or RNA sequences. By the binding of these nucleotides to their targets the transcription or translation of a single gene can be selectively inhibited. If that gene is responsible for a disease process then its down-regulation could result in a reversal of the clinical abnormalities. The cytoplasmic location of mRNA provides an easier target for oligodeoxinucleotides than DNA (see chapter by Hélène, this volume).

There are now several examples of antisense oligomers with anti-proliferative activity. These include c-myc in lymphoma cell lines containing abnormal transcripts [14]; N-myc in neurectodermal cell lines [15]; c-myb in colon adenocarcinoma [16]; type 1 regulatory subunit of the cAMP receptor protein kinase in k-ras transformed NIH3T3 cells [17], as well as neuroblastoma, leukaemia, breast, colon and gastric carcinoma cells; bcr-abl in chronic myeloid leukaemia blast cells [18]: and c-raf 1 in ras and raf NIH3T3 transformed cells [19].

Intriguingly, antisense oligonucleotides have been found to decrease tumorigenicity or the metastatic potential of several cell lines. A K-ras proto-oncogene in antisense orientation transduced into a small cell lung cancer cell line produced inhibition of K-ras expression and also the growth as tumours in nude mice.

There was no alteration in growth kinetics of the cell line *in vitro*. The antisense sequence to pre-proneurokinase significantly reduced the ability of murine melanoma cells to colonise lung. By contrast, if the antisense oligomer is designed to inhibit a putative metastasis suppressor gene such as E-cadherin, the resulting down-regulation renders the cells invasive [20]. These results demonstrate the power that antisense technology can display and the potential application it could have to manipulate abnormal growth.

Genetic Immunomodulation

It is clear from a decade of clinical trials that cytokines can have a very significant effect on tumour growth. However, these agents have been found to have highly toxic systemic effects and also an extremely short half-life *in vivo*. Many of the current prospects for gene therapy involve the vectoring of genes coding for these agents using cells that home specifically on tumours.

The anti-tumour immune response to the host can be improved by modifications of the immune system. Such modifications include the transfection of pleiotropic cytokine genes into the immune cells of the host or into tumour cells. It has now been demonstrated that the expression of cytokines in transfected cells can reduce their tumorigenicity and/or their metastatic potential. The anti-tumour response can be enhanced by the presence of cytotoxic lymphocytes, macrophages or antibodies which can in turn be induced by the expression of appropriate cytokine by tumour cells. In this way it may be possible to convert what would normally be a weakly immunogenic tumour eliciting only a minor response to a strongly immunogenic and therefore easily destroyed tumour. It has been demonstrated that the enhanced expression of major histocompatibility (MHC) molecules of both class I and II can be achieved either by the use of transfected cytokine genes or by direct MHC gene transfection.

The best characterised model so far has been the transfection of the tumour necrosis factor (TNF) gene into tumour infiltrating lymphocytes. TNF has produced very encouraging antitumour data in mice and yet its clinical results are extremely poor. This may reflect the dose limitation caused by its extreme toxicity in humans. Toxicity is common at doses above 8 micrograms per kilogram in man, whereas in mouse 400 micrograms per kilogram can be achieved. If a higher local concentration could be reached then perhaps the response rate to this interesting molecule might increase.

In the first study published last year it was demonstrated that in patients with melanoma tumour infiltrating lymphocytes (TIL) that had been transfected with the reporter gene (neomycin phosphotransferase) had actually localised in the tumour and continued to express foreign genes for up to 10 months after transfection [21]. Currently, a trial with TNF transfected cells is under way. The aim of this study is to evaluate the effects of the infusion of TNF-transfected TIL cells in 50 patients with melanoma. It has previously been demonstrated that TIL cells produce responses in up to 30% of melanoma patients. The results from this clinical trial should be available over the next few months.

Another approach to genetic immunomodulation is vaccine development. The human papilloma virus (HPV), particularly subtype 16, has been implicated in the aetiology of cervical cancer. Several recombinant vaccines expressing the nuclear proteins E6 or E7 have already demonstrated to reduce the subsequent development of HPV-related tumours in a variety of animals. Fibroblast-like cells transfected with HPV16 E7 genes have been used to immunise syngeneic mice [22]. Interestingly, it has been shown that these cells confer protection against tumorigenicity of HPV-16 E7-positive tumour cells in these animals.

Normal Tissue Protection

The production of cytotoxic drug resistant stem cells may be a mechanism by which normal cells could be protected from treatment-related toxicity, so allowing dose maximisation. The proposed transgenes can render stem cells resistant to certain specific drugs or confer to them more widespread multidrug resistance (by the expression of the MDR1 gene). The most encouraging study so far has clearly demonstrated methotrexate resistance *in vivo* after the implantation of murine haemopoetic stem cells transfected with the dihydrofolate reductase gene [23].

A currently exciting clinical area is the infusion of haemopoetic colony-stimulating factors (CSF) to restore chemotherapy-related bone marrow suppression in cancer patients. These molecules include granulocyte (G-CSF), macrophage (M-CSF), granulocyte-macrophage (GM-CSF), erythropoetin (EPO), diverse interleukins and a relatively uncharacterised stem cell factor. An alternative to infusion would be the genetic manipulation of normal bone marrow cells prior to chemotherapy. This may achieve a more continuous effect than the infusion of a drug with a short half-life. One study has demonstrated that the stable transfection of human G-CSF into fibroblasts *in vitro* successfully produced a neutrophilia when implanted into nude mice. The number of haemopoetic progenitor cells in the spleen was increased as well as in the bone marrow. The GM-CSF gene has also been transfected and expressed showing increased tolerance to a range of cytotoxic drugs [24]. The main problem currently is the low efficiency of gene insertion in stem cells. Current estimates show ranges from 10-20% in murine stem cells and only 1-5% in primates.

Drug Targeting

There are several potential genetic mechanisms for drug targeting. Virally-directed enzyme prodrug therapy (VDEPT) is based on the vector being specifically expressed in cells with a tissue or tumour marker, but not in normal cells. Table 2 shows examples where there is either tumour-specific transcription machinery or tissue specificity for the relevant genes in a host tissue which is not essential for survival.

The best example of VDEPT working *in vitro* comes from the discrimination of normal liver and hepatoma cells by the differential expression of vectors containing promoters for albumin and alphafetoprotein. In normal liver a herpes simplex thymidine kinase gene has been shown to be expressed when coupled to the albumin promoter but not when coupled to an alphafetoprotein promoter. The converse applies in hepatoma cells. Thymidine kinase converts the prodrug Ara-A

Table 2. Virally-directed enzyme prodrug therapy (VDEPT)

Marker	Tissue-tumour
CEA	GI, lung
AFP	hepatoma, teratoma
DOPA decarboxylase	SCLC, neurectoderm
NSE	SCLC
Amylase	pancreas
PSA	prostate
Calcitonin	thyroid (medullary)
Thyroglobulin	thyroid
PEM	breast
Villin	GI
erb B2	breast, GI
erb B3	breast, GI

Vector specifically expressed in cells with a tissue or tumour marker
Selectivity based on possession of appropriate transcriptional machinery by host cell

(vidarabine) which has minimal effects in normal cells, to Ara-AMP, Ara-ADP and Ara-ATP which are potent cytotoxics (Fig. 1).

Another similar prodrug system is the conversion of the antifungal 5-fluorocytosine to the cytotoxic drug 5-fluorouracil by cytosine deaminase driven off a selective promoter. A strategy for developing the 5-fluorouracil/VDEPT system in breast and gastrointestinal cancer is outlined in Figure 2. There are several steps for potential selectivity. The first is based on selective infection by the virus. This can be achieved by some form of targeting using immunoliposomes or a virus with predetermined tissue specificity. The second and perhaps most important selection is the expression of the vector only in the target cells with the appropriate transcription machinery.

Gene Replacement Therapy

It is now known that a variety of human tumours express upregulated oncogenes or down-regulated tumour suppressor genes. Mutants with defective function, both positive and negative, also coexist for both groups. There is now good evidence that *in vitro* reversion of malignant morphology can be achieved by a variety of different sequences, e.g., normal H-*ras*, K-*rev* and c-*jun*. Other sequences can increase the immunogenicity of

VDEPT

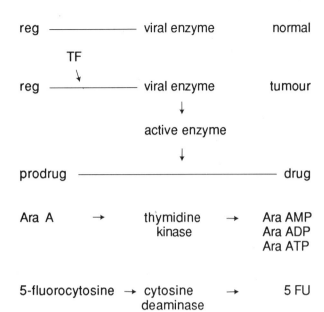

reg ——————— viral enzyme   normal

          TF
           ↓
reg ——————— viral enzyme   tumour
                    ↓
            active enzyme
                    ↓
prodrug ————————————————— drug

Ara A   →   thymidine   →   Ara AMP
                      kinase   Ara ADP
                                          Ara ATP

5-fluorocytosine → cytosine →   5 FU
                    deaminase

VDEPT

LTR ---- neo R ---- HSV - TK ---- AFP ---- LTR

LTR ---- neo R ---- HSV - TK ---- ALB ---- LTR

normal liver   ALB +   AFP -
hepatoma   ALB -   AFP +

Fig. 1. Virally directed enzyme prodrug therapy. The presence of the appropriate transcription factors in the host cell results in the production of the viral enzyme in the vector, so activating the prodrug. The best example of selective toxicity is the discrimination of normal liver and hepatoma cells by retroviral vectors containing alphafetoprotein (AFP) and albumin promotors. Normal liver cells are destroyed by the albumin vector and hepatoma cells by the construct containing the AFP promotor

tumour cells making them more susceptible to the cellular anti-tumoural response of the host. Further genes are able to selectively inhibit the metastatic potential of cells: nm23, ß-actin, fibronectin receptor, connexin and E-cadherin. Finally, there are genes with recognised tumour suppressor properties such as Rb and wild type p53.

obtain cytosine deaminase vector
                ↓
identify suitable promoter systems for selective expression in breast/GI cancer (erb B2, erb B3, PEM, villin)
                ↓
construct vector with relevant promoters
                ↓
check selective expression in high and low expressing cell lines
                ↓
assess kinetics and cytotoxicity with 5-fluorocytosine
                ↓
assess *in vivo* infectivity
                ↓
develop selective vector targeting immunoliposomes
                ↓
assess 5FU release kinetics *in vivo* PET
                ↓
phase I clinical trial

Fig. 2. Strategy for developing 5FU VDEPT system in breast and gastrointestinal cancer

The wild type p53 gene (WTp53) encodes a short half-life nuclear phosphoprotein with many properties consistent with tumour suppressor activity. It has been shown that WTp53 can promote cell differentiation as well as suppressing the proliferation rate of tumour-transfected cells. The expression of this gene can abolish tumorigenicity *in vivo* when such cells are placed in nude mice. The expression of wild type p53 but not mutant p53 has been shown to inhibit the cell proliferation of different human cell lines lacking p53 expression or expressing a mutated p53 allele. These include colorectal, osteosarcoma, glioblastoma and ovarian carcinoma cells [25]. p53 mutations have now been implicated as a late event in tumour progression in many human cancers and it may be possible to develop homologous recombination systems to insert functional p53 in place of the mutated gene.

The loss or inactivation of both retinoblastoma alleles has been observed in different types of tumours. These include retinoblastoma, breast cancer, small cell lung cancer, prostate, bladder, osteosarcoma and other soft tissue tumours [24]. Rb gene transfection into Rb-negative or Rb-mutated cells from retinoblastoma, osteosarcoma and prostate carcinoma lines can inhibit the malignant phenotype both *in vitro* and *in vivo*. The mechanisms by which this gene exerts its action are complex. There is evidence that p105 Rb acts as a transcription factor binding to DNA. Mutation, deletion or sequestration by adenovirus E1a, SV40 virus T and human papilloma virus type 16 E7 protein may result in a uncontrolled growth. The demonstration that the insertion of this gene in appropriate model systems can restore normal growth control provides an encouraging avenue for further development [26].

Another intriguing molecule is GC factor (GCF). This is the product of a gene that encodes a transcription factor that down-regulates the expression of certain genes associated with human cancer. *In vitro* assays have shown that this factor inhibits the transcription of EGF receptor, ß-actin and calcium-dependent protease by interacting with their promotors. This is due to its affinity for specific GC-rich sequences found in these and other regulatory sites [27]. The significance in cancer suppression *in vivo* remains to be elucidated. It may well act as a model system for studying down-regulation of growth by similar mechanisms.

The main problem with gene replacement therapy is the lack of suitable control technology for expression vectors. It is therefore unlikely that this strategy will have direct consequences in clinical care for at least 5 years.

Conclusions

There have been remarkable developments in our understanding of the molecular basis of human cancer. It is likely that this will continue to be enhanced as we learn more about the structure of the human genome and the mechanics of transcriptional control. Clearly, the discovery of a system of positively acting growth signals and negatively acting growth inhibitory signals working in parallel will lead to new rationally designed pharmacological agents active against cancer. Furthermore, by developing selective mechanisms to target-specific genes, completely new avenues for therapeutic endeavour will be open as we reach the end of this decade.

REFERENCES

1   Mastrangelo MJ, Schultz S, Kanem et al: Newer immunologic approaches to the treatment of patient with cancer. Sem Oncol 1988 (15):658-672
2   Smith KA: Interleukin 2: inception, inport and implications. Science 1988 (240):1169-70
3   Bishop JM: Molecular themes in oncogenesis. Cell 1991 (64):235-248
4   Slebos RT, Kiberlaan RE, Paledio O et al: K-ras oncogene activation as a prognostic marker in adenocarcinoma of the lung. New Engl J Med 1990 (323):561-565
5   Weatherall DJ: Gene therapy in perspective. Nature 1991 (349):255-276
6   Benvenisty N and Reshef L: Direct introduction of genes into rats and expression of the genes. Proc Natl Acad Sci USA 1986 (83):275-276
7   Ascadi G, Dicson G, Love DR, Jani A, Walsh FS, Gurusinghe A, Wolff JA, and Davies KE: Human dystrophin expression in mdx mice after intramuscular injection of DNA constructs. Nature 1991 (352):815-818
8   Geller AI, Keyomarsi K, Bryan J, and Pardee AB: An efficient deletion mutant packaging system for defective herpes simplex virus vectors: potential applications to human gene therapy and neuronal physiology. Proc Natl Acad Sci USA 1990 (87):8950-8954
9   Wu Ch, Wilson JM, and Wu Gy: Targeting genes: delivery and persistent expression of a foreign gene driven by mammalian regulatory elements in vivo. J Biol Chem 1989 (264):16985-16987
10   Kohn DB, Kantoff PW, Rglitis MA, McLachlin JR, Moen RC et al: Retroviral mediated gene transfer into mamalian cells. Blood 1987 (13):285-298
11   Temin HM: Overview of biological effects of addition of DNA molecules to cells. J. Med Virol 1990 (31):13-17
12   Johnson P, Gray D, Mowat M, and Benchimol S: Expression of wild-type p53 is not compatible with continued growth of p53-negative tumor cells. Mol Cell Biol 1991 (11):1-11
13   Miller AD: Retrovirus packaging cells. Human Gene Ther 1990 (1):5-14
14   McManaway ME, Neckers LM, Loke SL, Al Nasser AA, Redner RL et al: Tumour specific inhibition of lymphoma growth by an antisense oligodesoxynucleotide. Lancet 1990 (335):808-811
15   Whitesell L, Rosolen A, and Neckers LM: Episome-generated N-myc antisense RNA restricts the differentiation potential of primitive neuroectodermal cell lines. Mol Cell Biol 1991:1360-1370
16   Melani C, Rivoltini L, Parmiani G, Calabretta B, Colombo MP: Inhibition of proliferation by c-myb antisense oligodeoxynucleotides in colon adenocarcinoma cell lines that express c-myb. Cancer Res 1991 (51):2897-2901
17   Cho-Chung YS, Clair T, Tortora G, Yokozaki H and Pepi S: Supression of malignancy targeting the intracellular signal transducing proteins of cAMP: the use of site selective cAMP analogs antisense strategy and gene transfer. Life Sci 1991 (48):1123-1132
18   Szczylik C, Skorski T, Nicolaides NC, Manzella L, Malaguarnera L, Venturelli D, Gewirtz AM, Calabretta B: Selective inhibition of leukemia cell proliferation by BCR-ABL antisense oligodeoxynucleotides. Science 1991 (253):562-568
19   Kolch W, Heidecker G, Lloyd P and Rapp UR: Raf-1 protein kinase is required for growth of induced NIH/313 cells. Nature 1991 (349):426-428
20   Vleminck K, Vakaet L, Mareel M, Fiers W, Van Roy F: Genetic manipulation of E-Cadherin expression by epithelial tumor cells reveals an invasion suppressor role. Cell 1991 (66):107-119
21   Rosenberg SA, Albersold P, Cornetta K, Kasid A, Morgan RA et al: Gene transfer into humans-immunotherapy of patients with advanced melanoma, using tumor-infiltrating lymphocytes modified by retroviral gene transduction. N Engl J Med 1990 (323):570-578
22   Chen L, Thomas EK, Hu SL, Hellstrom I, Hellstrom KE: Human papilloma virus type 16 nucleoprotein E7 is a tumour rejection antigen. Proc Natl Acad Sci USA 1991 (88):110-114
23   Corey CA, Desilva AD, Holland CA, Williams DA: Serial transplantation of Methotrexate-resistance bone marrow: protection of murine recipients from drug toxicity by progency of transduced stem cells. Blood 1990 (75):337-343
24   Keith WN, Brown R, and Pragnell IB: Retrovirus mediated transer and expression of GM-CSF in haematopoietic cells. Br J Cancer 1990 (62):388-394
25   Mercer WE, Shields MT, Lin D, Appella E, and Ulrich SJ: Growth suppression induced by wild-type p53 protein is accompanied by selective down-regulation of proliferating-cell nuclear antigen expression. Proc Natl Acad Sci USA 1991 (88):1958-1962
26   Huang HJS, Yee JK, Shew JY, Chen PL, Bookstein R, Friedmann T et al: Suppression of the neoplastic phenotype by replacement of the RB gene in human cancer cells. Science 1988 (242):1563-1566
27   Johnson A, Kageyama R, Popescu NC and Pastan I: Expression and chromosomal localisation of the human transcriptional repressor GCF. J Biol Chem (in press)

Membrane and Signal Transduction Targets

John A. Hickman

The Cancer Research Campaign Molecular and Cellular Pharmacology Group, Department of Physiological Sciences, University of Manchester, Manchester, M13 9PT, United Kingdom

Recently, a torrent of biochemical and biological discoveries has more precisely begun to define the nature of the malignant phenotype. These findings present a formidable challenge to drug discovery teams. How can this knowledge be harnessed and the approach emulated? Sadly, the elegance and precision of some of the insights provided by molecular and cellular biologists have not yet been matched by the efforts of medicinal chemists and pharmacologists. It is both disappointing and frustrating that the anticancer drugs showing clinical promise in 1991 are still crude cell poisons, not dissimilar from those which exist in the current pharmacopoeia. How might progress be made?

The task ahead for the anticancer drug discoverer is difficult. First, cancer is a complex disease and its multistep nature begs the question as to whether targeting a single drug to a single locus can ever be successful. And, whilst the molecular biologists have provided stunning insights into, for example, the intricacies of the control of gene expression at the molecular and cellular level and how it may be subverted by the aberrant expression of certain genes, their studies have been essentially, and sensibly, reductionist in nature. A major criticism of their work might be that it has sometimes failed to integrate aspects of tumour biology, given its heterogeneity and instability, or to take account of tumour host interactions. The hapless pharmacologist must wrestle with this problem: how to meld reductionist knowledge with the ultimate goal of interfering with a complex pathology *in vivo*. How to identify molecular targets as templates for new, modulatory molecules, and then how to test for their potential efficacy in a setting representative of a growing tumour, which has arisen from a number of genetic changes. At each of these levels, the biochemical, the cellular and the tumour *in situ*, the activity of a new antitumour drug will essentially reflect the appropriateness of the screen which attempts to model the "real" situation.

Despite these concerns there are many new approaches being initiated which absorb the recent understanding of the molecular biology of cancer. One of the emerging and exciting frameworks for the potential discovery of new antitumour drugs is the growing understanding of the events at the surface of the cell which initiate cell division [1,2]. The identification of growth factors, their receptors, and the cascade of intracellular events which follows their interaction presents a plethora of potential targets for the pharmacologist. It is at this locus, the cell membrane, that the majority of pharmacological agents outside the anticancer pharmacopoeia exert their activity. It seems reasonable to expect that intervention at this locus may also modulate the control of cell division and other processes of importance in the malignant phenotype. This idea seems all the more rational given that the activity of the products of a number of oncogenes, which are suggested to play a role in the subversion of growth control, is exerted at the cell membrane [2-4] (Fig. 1). These genes variously encode for growth factors, growth factor receptor-like molecules which appear to be activated without ligand binding and putative elements of the signal transduction machinery such as GTP-binding proteins and kinases. It is important to note that growth factors and the cytokines provide not only sig-

Oncogenes

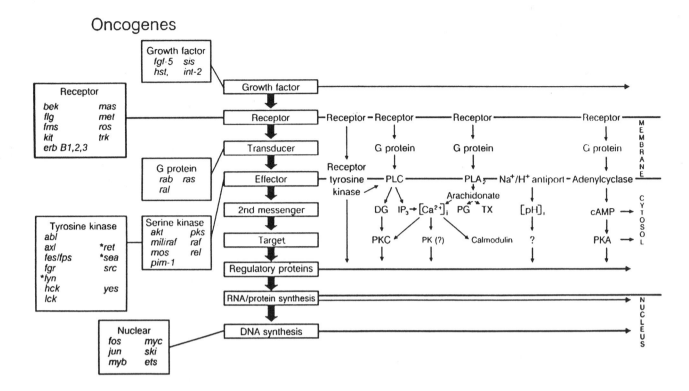

Fig. 1. The hierarchy of the cell signalling cascade and the involvement of oncogenes in the cascade (reproduced by permission of Dr Garth Powis)

nals for mitogenesis but also signals which may coordinately link growth *with* differentiation and the subsequent loss of proliferative potential. Additionally, some growth factors appear to provide signals for cell survival, and it is possible that these may be quite distinct from those stimulating mitogenesis. This topic is discussed below.

The chapter introduces some of the key components of membrane biochemistry involved in growth control whilst reviewing the actions of agents affecting these processes. It discusses some of the novel strategies that have been initiated and it describes some of the new molecules which are targeted at the membrane. It does not survey the effects of existing drugs on membrane function. The novel drugs, with an unproven clinical efficacy, inhibit either growth factor binding or growth factor receptor activation (particularly the stimulation of tyrosine kinase activity), second messenger generation or the activity of other protein kinases. In addition, some potentially new targets at the cell membrane are suggested as being ripe for consideration.

One of these is membrane-extracellular matrix interactions, another the domains of certain proteins (SH2 and SH3) which couple cell membrane proteins in signal cascades. The biological end points of these actions are considered and the chapter closes with a few caveats to pharmacologists and medicinal chemists attracted to study the potential for the modulation of membrane-associated biochemistry, a biochemistry which clearly is a critical component of the control of cellular activity.

Growth Factor Antagonists

The signals for growth, differentiation and survival are provided by growth factors and cytokines emanating from, potentially, autocrine, paracrine or endocrine loops. In tumour cells the expression of these factors in an autocrine manner probably reflects the primitive stage in which the cell has become blocked in its differentiation. This supports the notion that tumour cells have uncoupled their proliferation from the normal process of differentiation, giving rise to daughter cells which are relatively undifferentiated and which maintain their proliferative potential. What advances have been made in inhibiting these autocrine signals?

The focus of much work in this area has been on the inhibition of bombesin-stimulated growth of small cell lung cancer (SCLC) and an account of some of this work provides a good example of the progress and pitfalls of these early attempts to generate new types of growth inhibitor. SCLC cells secrete a number of neuropeptides and growth factors including bombesin (or its mammalian homologue gastrin releasing peptide, grp) [5] and it was reasonably presumed that inhibition of bombesin binding to its receptor would inhibit SCLC growth. Indeed, early results showed that an anti-bombesin antibody inhibited growth of SCLC cell lines *in vitro* and the growth of a xenograft in mice [6]. Subsequent problems with this antibody arose in phase I clinical trials, reputedly because of the production of anti-idiotype antibodies. These have the potential to act as bombesin receptor agonists. The second approach has been the synthesis of peptide antagonists of bombesin. The elegant studies of Rozengurt and colleagues have used Swiss 3T3 cells to establish the nature of the signalling cascade stimulated by bombesin and other mitogens such as vasopressin and bradykinin. They reported that these act through distinct receptors to elevate intracellular calcium and that bombesin acts via a G protein [7]. This is supported by the evidence from the cloning of the bombesin receptor [8] which showed that the receptor is one of the super-family of receptors with 7 transmembrane spanning segments [9]. The bombesin-stimulated rises in intracellular calcium in Swiss 3T3 cells acted as the basis for the selection of a range of specific and non-specific (inhibiting a calcium rise induced by other ligands) bombesin antagonists by Woll and Rozengurt. These were then assayed against a number of SCLC cells stimulated by grp [10,11]. The compounds ranged from [Leu^{13}-*psi*(CH$_2$NH) Leu^{14}]bombesin, which was a specific antagonist of bombesin, to substance P analogues, such as [Arg^6,DTrp^{7,9},MePhe^8] substance P(6-11), which was non-specific. Although each was found to be an inhibitor of the grp-stimulated rise in calcium, the non-specific compounds for the bombesin receptor were more effective inhibitors of SCLC growth [11, 12]. This result is not altogether surprising, given that the cells contain multiple growth factor receptors but it suggests that efficacy can only be achieved at the expense of selectivity - an old problem.

It is unlikely that the stimulus for proliferation, differentiation and survival signals will be provided by one ligand binding to one receptor. It is also possible that cross-talk between receptors may compensate for the loss of signal at a single locus. If this is the case, then clearly growth factor antagonists may not emerge as useful single agents, but this has to be established by experiments in other systems which parallel those above.

Tyrosine Kinase Inhibitors

The regulation of cellular activity by the action of protein kinases is predominantly mediated through changes in the phosphorylated status of serine and threonine residues. The activity of many growth and differentiating factors is instead associated with the phosphorylation of tyrosine residues via the activities of their transmembrane spanning receptors [13]. Additionally, membrane-associated proto-oncogene and viral oncogene products, such as *src*, *yes*, and *abl*, possess tyrosine kinase activity [14]. The activity of protein tyrosine kinases associated with the products of many oncogenes which are putative growth factor receptors (*erb B-2*, *fms*, *met*, *ros*, *kit*, *trk*, *ret*) has alerted medicinal chemists to the possibility of selectively inhibiting this class of kinase.

Several reports have been made of the activity of both synthetic and natural products as inhibitors of tyrosine kinases [15-20] and some of these compounds have then been used as "lead" compounds in synthetic chemistry programmes aimed at producing more potent and specific inhibitors. For example, Glossman et al. [21] reported that the flavone quercetin (Fig. 2) was an inhibitor of tyrosine phosphorylation by the transforming

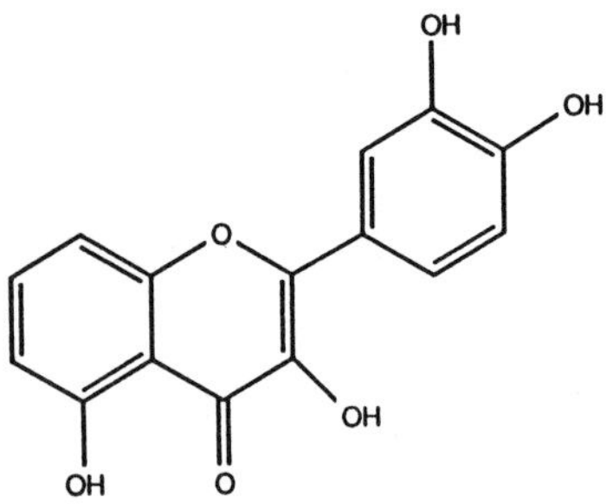

Quercetin 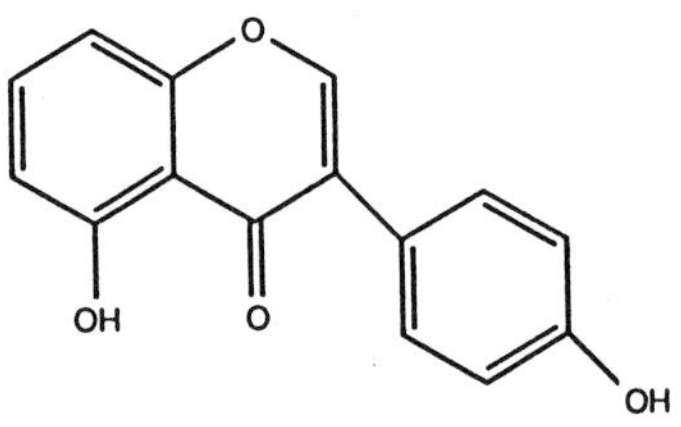   Genestein

Fig. 2. The structures of flavone and isoflavone inhibitors of protein tyrosine kinases

protein kinase pp60[src] but inhibited cAMP-dependent protein kinase less potently. This finding of some specificity of inhibition proved intriguing when it was later shown to be competitive with respect to ATP (half maximal inhibition at 3-4µM) [22]. This is intriguing because the ATP binding site across the whole family of protein kinases is highly conserved [23] so that one would not expect any such specificity.

The isoflavone genestein (Fig. 2) was reported to be a much more specific inhibitor of the tyrosine kinase family although its potency resembled that of quercetin [24]. Inhibition of pp60[src], pp110[gag-fes] and the epidermal growth factor (EGF) receptor kinase was competitive with respect to ATP but IC_{50}s of the order of 6-7µM against the tyrosine kinases were markedly lower than the values (>100µM) for inhibition of protein kinase C, 5'-nucleotidase and cAMP protein kinase. Interestingly, genestein was not found to be an inhibitor of p40, a tyrosine kinase activity associated with normal thymocytes [25], a finding which holds promise for the potential specificity of the flavones and isoflavones. Ogawara et al. [26] investigated the activity of genestein and a number of other flavones on the growth of Rous sarcoma-transformed cells but found no correlation between growth inhibition and their activity as kinase inhibitors. We found essentially the same with a series of synthetic flavones active against the Abelson tyrosine kinase: there was no correlation with growth inhibition of Abelson transformed 3T3 cells compared to wild-type 3T3 cells [27]. However, we found a 4'-aminoflavone to be extremely toxic to the transformed cells in comparison to their normal counterparts and we were interested to see a recent report [28] of a 4'-aminoflavone as the most potent (IC_{50} = 1µM) of a series of flavones tested as inhibitors of p56[lck], a T-cell tyrosine kinase related to src. It is likely that results from our laboratory with a 4'-aminoflavone indicate that targets other than abl are responsible for growth inhibition. This problem of correlating enzyme inhibition data to growth inhibition of cells transformed with the appropriate enzyme is a theme which emerges strongly in studies of other inhibitors, as related below.

A group of thiazolidine-diones were reported to have superior selectivity to genestein [29] and, most interestingly, showed potent inhibition of the tyrosine kinase activity of the src protein, with mixed kinetics of inhibition with respect to ATP, but little inhibition of the highly homologous abl protein. Clearly, a range of kinases have to be tested when first screening these types of inhibitors.

Although there has been much activity in the flavone field, the basis of their action as competitive inhibitors of ATP is less attractive than the design of selective agents which are competitive with respect to the substrate. Here, the lead compound has been the natural product erbstatin (Fig. 3), which was claimed to be non-competitive with ATP but competitive with peptide in assays of the EGF receptor protein tyrosine kinase [30]. However, erbstatin now has been shown to be less selective than first claimed, inhibiting protein kinase C with an IC_{50} of 20µM. This inhibition was competitive with respect to ATP [31]. The authors query whether some of the

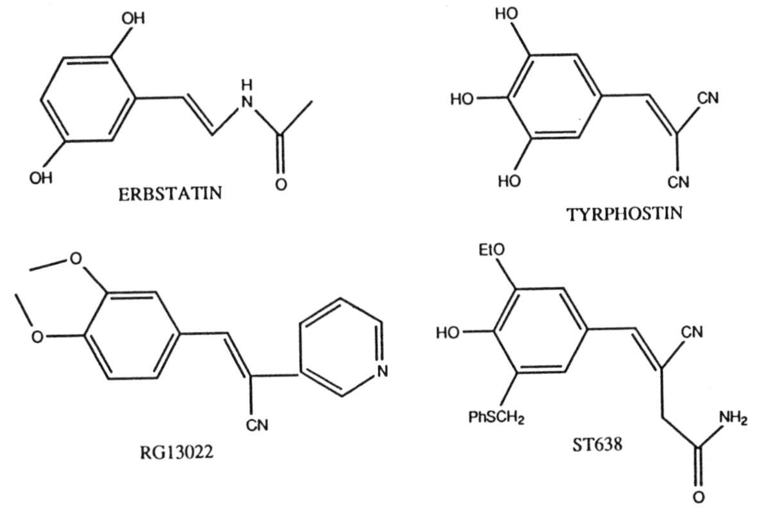

Fig. 3. Structures of erbstatin analogues: the tyrphostins and 4-hydroxycinnamide derivatives

inhibition of tumour cell growth reported for erbstatin was actually due to inhibition of tyrosine kinase activity [32].

This type of controversy spills over to the mechanism of action of the most potent series of erbstatin analogues, the tyrphostins (Fig. 3) [33]. The tyrphostins are a series of substituted benzylidene-malononitriles which showed a 100 to 800-fold differential inhibition of the tyrosine kinase activity of the EGF receptor and the insulin receptor. Most importantly, the activity of the compounds against the growth of an EGF-stimulated clone of A431 cells was reversible [34] and shown to be competitive with respect to substrate [35]. This aspect of the mechanism of tyrosine kinase inhibitors is discussed further, below. Extensive synthetic chemistry by Levitski and his colleagues has produced a series of compounds with some selective activity for the HER1 (EGF receptor kinase) and related HER 2 (erb-B2, neu) protein [36]. The expression of erb-B2 is an independent indicator of poor prognosis in breast cancer [37].

There are conflicting reports as to whether these apparently highly selective inhibitors of substrate binding [35] actually modulate cell growth because they inhibit tyrosine kinase activity. Thus, Faaland et al. [38] showed that a tyrphostin could relieve the growth inhibition imposed by EGF in a clone of A431 cells which greatly overexpress the EGF receptor. However, the relief of EGF-imposed growth inhibition in this clone was not due to any inhibition of EGF receptor-associated tyrosine kinase activity. A tyrphostin (RG-13022) has been shown recently to inhibit the growth of a xenograft in vivo, although the authors accepted that the protocol for achieving an increase in the life-span of the animals depended on multiple dosing schedules that had to be initiated at the same time as tumour transplant [39]. Evidence was presented in this paper that the compound inhibited the autophosphorylation of the EGF receptor in cell free extracts taken from EGF receptor transfected NIH 3T3 cells, and also in whole cells after an overnight incubation. What is not clear is whether this inhibition was specific and correlatable with growth inhibition and no data were presented on changes of phosphorylation status of the cells in vivo.

The tyrphostin story has rather overshadowed the interesting activity of structurally similar 4-hydroxycinnamamide derivatives [40]. One of these compounds, ST 638 (Fig. 3) showed discriminatory inhibition amongst a range of oncogene proteins. Kinetic analysis showed these compounds to be competitive with an exogenous substrate, with a Ki of 2μM.

Despite the caveats regarding some of these compounds, further development will hopefully see the emergence of a receptor-mediated inhibitor of tumour cell growth. It is most important that authors attempt to validate the implied claims that inhibition of tumour cell growth in vivo is really due to a specific biochemical effect of the compound. Whether these compounds should be screened as potential antiproliferatives is an important corollary: antibodies to a sequence in the tyrosine kinase pp60[src] inhibited membrane ruffling in KB cells [41], and temperature switching of temperature-sensitive mutants to the non-permissive temperature did not result in a loss of cell viability [42]. More subtle end points may be appropriate to the role of the tyrosine kinase family in control of not only proliferation, but also differentiation and survival.

Receptor-Transducer Coupling: SH2 Domains as Potential Targets

The binding of a growth factor or cytokine to a transmembrane receptor initiates a series of events which result in metabolic changes inside the cell. Events occurring at the outer leaflet of the membrane must therefore be coupled in some way to the machinery on the inner leaflet. The biochemical determinants of this "coupling" process are just emerging and the story is one which seems eminently exploitable by the drug discoverer because it provides targets which have intrinsically high specificity associated with them. When the EGF receptor, and other receptors, become stimulated they become associated with several proteins, including phospholipase C, p21^{ras} GTPase-activating protein (GAP), *src* and *src*-like tyrosine kinases and phosphatidylinositol-3'-kinase. Although different in function, each of these associated proteins contain conserved non-catalytic domains called src homology regions or SH regions 2 and 3 [2,43]. It is suggested that these domains are involved in the interactions of proteins to receptor tyrosine kinases. The SH2 regions appear to control the coupling of proteins involved in signal transduction and are attracted to areas of tyrosine phosphorylation on the membrane receptor. Autophosphorylation sites at tyrosine residues on membrane proteins attract SH2 motifs expressed in these other proteins so that inhibition of tyrosine kinase activity (and autophosphorylation) by the drugs described above will, potentially, prevent receptor coupling and signal transduction. A scheme describing this idea is shown in Figure 4.

The different responses to a growth factor observed in different cells appears to be regulated by the repertoire of SH2 interactions offered by each cell. SH2 sequences have well conserved domains separated by variable domains which may act as "hinges". The

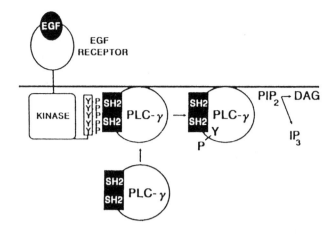

Fig. 4. The possible binding of SH2 sequences in PLCγ to the autophosphorylation sites in the EGF receptor. (Reproduced with permission from ref. 43)

sequence differences in each protein are considered to impart a specificity of binding and the sequence motifs involved in the active domains have been suggested to be only short runs of amino acids since they bind after denaturation of the whole protein (shown below). This suggests that these sequences should be easy to mimic using synthetic peptides. It should also be easy for their conformation to be determined so that synthetic strategies can be initiated to provide small molecule inhibitors of undesirable SH2 couplings - for example of the *erb*-B2 receptor protein with whatever its down-stream effector may be.

c-Src   **WYFGKIT**...RRE...sERILLnPeNpr.....
GTFLVRESETTK.GAYcLSVsDF.DnaKGlnn**VKHYKIR**
KLDsGGFYYITSRtQ...FSSQqTLVaYYSKhAD..GLCh..R
LTnV

c-Abl   **WYHGPVS**..RNA...AEY.LLSSGIN......
GSFLYRESESSP.G.QR.SISLRYE...G.**RVYHYRI**.N
TasDGKlYVSsESR...FNTLAELVHHHSTVAD..GLITT...L
HYPA

PLC-Y1N   **WFHGKL**gagRdgrhiAER.LLtEYCiETGA
pD**GSFLVRESETF**v.GDYTLSF..WRn...G.**KVQHCRI**
hSRqDaGtpkFFLTDNLvFdSLYDLITHYqqVPRRCNEFEM.
.RLSEPV

Alternatively, in the *src* protein the SH2 sequence may bind to its own C-terminal region of tyrosine autophosphorylation (Fig. 5) and

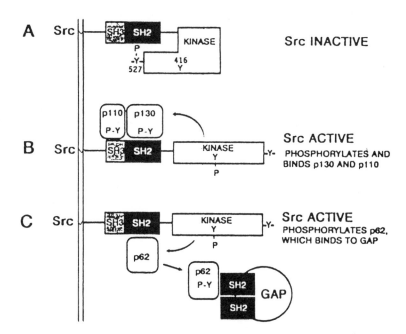

Fig. 5. Possible interactions of the *src* SH2 domains with the autophosphorylation site at Tyr527 which is a negative regulatory site, so as to "mask" activity. Dephosphorylation of Tyr527 leads to a conformational change which exposes autophosphorylation sites now capable of interaction with the SH2 domains of other proteins in the cascade. (Reproduced with permission from ref. 43)

hence act as an autoinhibitor. Synthesis of a drug which mimics this intramolecular SH2 binding should inhibit the activity of this oncogene product [44]. Thus far, there have been no reports of such strategies.

Inhibition of Second Messenger Function

Inositol Derivatives

Surprisingly little has emerged into the published literature of attempts to inhibit the signalling processes initiated by the inositol lipids. The highly conserved bifurcating pathway of signal generation which results from the breakdown of phosphatidylinositol-4,5-bisphosphate to 1,4,5-inositol trisphosphate and a diacylglycerol [45] does not suggest itself as a target for selective intervention because of its conserved nature. Agonists of the water soluble, calcium releasing inositol-1,4,5-trisphosphate have been reported which utilised 2' position substitutions but these were not assayed for their activities against transformed cells but rather as inhibitors of the putatively inactivating 3'kinase [46]. Stable analogues of inositol 1,4,5-trisphosphate which contained a phosphorothioate linkage in different positions on the

inositol sugar have been shown to be agonists for calcium release [47], but the role of such compounds as antagonists for cell growth has not been evaluated. With respect to the possible selectivity of these compounds, data suggesting that there are different "pools" of inositol phospholipids which might be differentially activated by different ligand-receptor interactions [48], allows speculation that selective modulation of mobilisation might be possible.

The possibilities of selective intervention of inositol signalling are opened by the findings that a number of protein tyrosine kinases, the activity of which is elevated in transformed cells, are associated with a phosphatidylinositol 3'-kinase [2]. The phosphatidylinositol-3'-phosphates are not substrates for hydrolysis by phospholipase C and instead perform an as yet ill-defined role in regulating cell growth and differentiation. It is clear from sight-directed mutagenesis experiments that failure to achieve a coupling between the transforming tyrosine kinases and the 3'-inositol kinase abrogates transformation.

Powis et al. [49] have synthesised a series of 3'-*myo*-inositol analogues for evaluation of their effects on growth and signalling. Inhibition of growth was assessed in a pair of NIH 3T3 cell lines, one of which had been transformed with the oncogene v-*sis*. Differential activities were discovered. For example, D-3-deoxy-3-azido-*myo*-inositol showed a >1,200-fold greater toxicity to the transformed cell line and its activity could be diminished by co-incubation with *myo*-inositol. However, potency of many of the analogues was low, with IC_{50}s generally in the mM range and the mechanism of growth inhibition remains speculative, with no secure evidence that the 3'-kinase was the target. Nevertheless, this study heralds a new approach to antimetabolite therapy which may provide useful agents in the future and should also provide useful research tools for the dissection of these complex signalling pathways.

Protein Kinase C

Another highly conserved player in the cascade following receptor mediated activation of cells is protein kinase C, sometimes said to be the enzyme at the "crossroads" of many activation pathways. Protein kinase C is activated by diacylglycerols and the activation process is followed by a period of down-regulation after enzyme cleavage. This down-regulation may play as important a role in the control of cellular activity as the activation process itself. There is thus a temporal aspect to the role of protein kinase C's activity in the cell. The search for inhibitors of this family of enzymes has been the subject of an excellent review [50] as has the enzyme's role in malignant cells [51]. Once again, the question of whether selective intervention at this target is possible remains to be determined. The argument in favour of this possibility rests on the fact that protein kinase C is a family of enzymes, the members of which are differentially and heterogeneously expressed according to cell type. Not only might expression be differential but in response to extracellular signals, the sub-species are down-regulated at different rates [52].

Of the various modulators of protein kinase C activity with potential antitumour activity, the bryostatins have received most attention, and bryostatin 1 has been entered into a phase I clinical trial in the UK. The activity of this complex molecule (both in terms of its chemistry and its biology) was first discovered in the standard murine screening models [53] and reports of its *in vivo* activity continue to appear [54].

Aspects of the biological activity of the bryostatins are worth brief review here not least because bryostatin 1 has entered clinical trial. The trial raises a number of interesting questions. The drug has, as will be described below, a complex and unresolved mechanism of action and it is therefore difficult to know how to use it in the clinic. Is it appropriate to conduct a classical phase I trail which attempts to determine the maximum tolerated dose and then treat patients at a dose just below this? Such an approach would not be appropriate in the trial of, say, a new neuroleptic. Should a modulator of cellular signalling be treated in a way different from a standard cytotoxic drug? Analysis of its effects on chronic myelogenous leukaemic cells suggests it to be cytotoxic because of the induction of Tumour Necrosis Factor [55]. Direct effects, to bring about cytostasis, were observed against fresh human acute non-lymphocytic leukaemia cells, with 3-4 logs. of inhibition of cloning potential, whereas the effect of bryostatin 1 on normal elements of haematopoiesis was to stimulate CFU-GMs in the presence of rGM-CSF [56]. This differential of activity is clearly very attractive. How might it be accounted for? The biochemical effects of bryostatin 1 are paradoxical since it binds to and activates protein kinase C yet blocks the actions of phorbol esters and, in HL-60 cells, blocks the differentiation promoting effects of TPA without itself affecting differentiation [57]. Moreover, in A549 human lung carcinoma cells bryostatin 1 abolished its own inhibition of DNA synthesis *in vitro* as its concentration was elevated [58]! From a number of such paradoxical results, a consensus hypothesis is emerging which suggests that these properties may be explained by differential effects on members of the protein kinase C isozymes. For example, the activation of protein kinase C in HL-60 human promyelocytic leukaemia cells does not engage differentiation but instead inhibits phorbol ester-induced differentiation (presumably also mediated by the activation of protein kinase C). This divergent response appears to correlate with the activation by bryostatin 1 of a protein kinase C-like activity in the nucleus which may be PKC β_{II}. Phorbol dibutyrate translocated both PKCα **and** PKCβ_{II} [59] whereas bryostatin 1

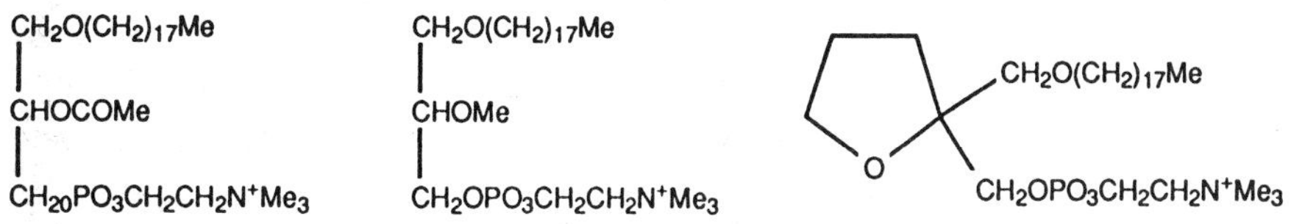

CH₂O(CH₂)₁₇Me
|
CHOCOMe
|
CH₂OPO₃CH₂CH₂N⁺Me₃

PAF

CH₂O(CH₂)₁₇Me
|
CHOMe
|
CH₂OPO₃CH₂CH₂N⁺Me₃

ET-18-OMe

CH₂O(CH₂)₁₇Me

CH₂OPO₃CH₂CH₂N⁺Me₃

SRI 62-834

Fig. 6. The structures of platelet activating factor and two ether lipids, currently in clinical trial

was selective for the translocation of PKCβ$_{II}$. It is this type of selectivity that should establish protein kinase C as a target capable of selective manipulation, even if bryostatin 1 itself does not prove to have therapeutic efficacy.

Ether Lipids

The antitumour ether lipids and structurally related drugs have been the subject of a very good recent review [60]. The first ether lipids were analogues of lysophosphatidylcholine and are also analogues of platelet activating factor (Fig. 6) [61].

The *in vivo* activity of these agents [60,61], their extraordinary *in vitro* selectivity for leukaemic cell lines compared to a non-tumourigenic stem cell-like line (FDCP mix A4 cells) (Fig. 7) and their novel mechanism of action has promoted the clinical trial of 4 such compounds. Berdel [60] has expressed doubts regarding the potential clinical efficacy of these compounds. As lipids, the compounds are heavily plasma protein-bound and the reduction of efficacy may well be due to pharmacokinetic limitations. Some imaginative chemistry may resolve this problem.

Despite reservations about their current clinical efficacy, albeit in phase 1 trials which aim to determine toxicity, not therapeutic effect, studies of the mechanism of action of the ether lipids have presented us with a unique result with respect to the selectivity of this class of compound - these are truly "antitumour compounds" (Fig. 7). The biochemical basis for this phenomenal selectivity may provide clues as to how some inherent difference between a stem cell and a leukaemic cell might be exploited in some other way, if not by the ether lipids themselves. The work of Bazill and Dexter [62] has suggested that the ether lipids are taken up

by an active endocytotic mechanism and that the differential accumulation of the compounds accounts for their selectivity. Although these data are based on short-term (24-48h) measurements of membrane integrity, the modulation of this acute toxicity by inhibitors of endocytosis such as quinidine reduced the rate of membrane breakdown.

The question of whether the ether lipids act in a mechanical way to disrupt membranes, in a manner dependent upon their differential rates of accumulation, or whether they have subtle effects on cell signalling cascades, remains open to debate. In our recent experiments, and those of others which aim to

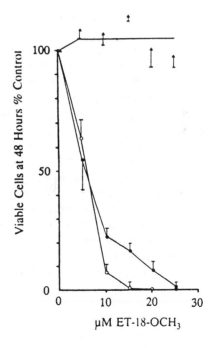

Fig. 7. The selective effect of the ether lipid Et-18-OCH3 against a non-tumourigenic murine haematopoietic stem cell line FDCP-A4 Mix and two leukaemic cell lines HL-60 and WEHI-3B. Viable counts were recorded by estimation of trypan blue exclusion. KEY: l = WEHI-3B cells ; s = FDCP-A4 Mix cells; m = HL-60 cells (Reproduced with permission from ref. 62)

assess the role of changes in intracellular calcium induced by ether lipids [63,64], toxicity is only observed when the cell membranes become leaky to calcium indicators [65]. On balance, it would appear that these agents do not have subtle effects on cell signalling at effective concentrations required for cell killing and that efficacy is dependent on selective accumulation.

The Extracellular Matrix: Signals Which Induce Differentiation

It is essential that the major cancers in man, the carcinomas, be targeted for chemotherapy. The effective coupling of growth and the highly organised differentiation of epithelial tissues depend upon the presence of an extracellular matrix, more specifically a basement membrane which consists of collagen IV, fibronectin and laminin [66]. Laminin anchors the basal lamina to the cell surface. Laminin, and other matrix components, interact with a family of integrin membrane receptors but how binding to these receptors may change gene expression to signal for the maintenance of organised tissue architecture and function is unclear. The disorganised growth of carcinomas may in part be due to the failure of the cells to receive or respond to signals provided at the membrane by components of a basal lamina via these integrin receptors.

The elegant work of Bissell and colleagues [67] has shown that mammary epithelial cells without an extracellular matrix become squamous and undifferentiated in morphology and fail to express gene products typical of the functional mammary gland, such as the milk protein whey acidic protein. When these cells were grown on components of a basement membrane, morphological and functional differentiation occurred, with not only the expression of milk protein but its secretion into the media from polarised epithelial structures. Differentiation of this type is also associated with a decrease in the fraction of cells with proliferative potential.

Our own studies have shown that anaplastic murine colon adenocarcinoma cells will undergo significant differentiation when grown on floating rafts of type 1 collagen [68], but a large proportion of the cells remained anaplastic and maintained their proliferative potential. What is it that allows some of these tumour cells to undergo terminal differentiation and why do some not respond? An understanding of the signals generated by components of the extracellular matrix, and presumably transduced by receptors like the integrin receptor, may provide targets for drug intervention which are not related to proliferative biochemistry.

Caveats and Conclusions

This chapter has reviewed some of the developments in the area of membrane-active antitumour drugs. Many aspects of recent progress have not been tackled, for example the interesting work on suramin and its inhibition of growth factor-receptor interactions [69], and it is certain that the field will expand further in the next few years. So-called "membrane targets" now encompass a wide variety of processes integrating the cascades of signals which control proliferation and differentiation. Most of the active drug molecules interact with membrane-associated proteins. Instead of thinking of these targets as being somehow completely different from those exploited by chemotherapists in the past, they should perhaps be considered as novel targets for new types of "antimetabolites".

There is, however, a major caveat to some of the current approaches. One of the major goals of the drug discoverer is to find agents which will inhibit the growth of the common solid tumours. These are generally low growth fraction tumours and so many cells are not expressing proliferative biochemistry during the window of time in which drugs are present. The new framework for drug discovery provided by the biochemistry of signal cascades is descriptive of events which control proliferation; it is a new biochemistry in comparison to that of the synthesis and replication of DNA, but nevertheless it is still a biochemistry of events which occur in proliferating cells. We are therefore faced with the potential of some new and exciting molecules which may have the same spectrum of activity as present drugs because they have the potential to affect dividing cells only.

Cancer is a disease not only of aberrant proliferation (if it was one might expect more high growth fraction tumours) but of aberrant differentiation. The view of the cancer cell as one in which differentiation (and the ability to senesce) has been blocked may be useful [70]. The uncoupling of differentiation from proliferation in the tumour cell suggests that the oncogenic proteins which usurp signal pathways for differentiation may be more appropriate targets for drug design. The task of teasing apart the signals for proliferation from those for differentiation (often with many features conserved) has only recently begun. The signals which are initiated by the binding of cytokines such as GM-CSF to their receptors, and which clearly drive differentiation are almost completely unknown [71, 72]. There is therefore the prospect of a new and more appropriate framework in which to perform drug hunting.

Finally, the growth and normal homeostasis of organ size depends upon the tight maintenance of a balance between cell gain, via proliferation, and cell loss via terminal differentiation (with loss of proliferative potential) and cell death. It is becoming clear that a feature of tumour cell growth which has not received sufficient attention is that of tumour cell dynamics: the balance between the rates of cell loss and gain may be aberrant, with insufficient cell loss. What is known about this cell loss? In normal tissues this appears to be by the process of apoptosis, or programmed cell death. If a programmed cell death is a phenotypically determined characteristic of cells one must ask what signals might be involved in initiating and modulating it. Could this signalling process be usurped by the oncogenic process? And might it not be attractive to look for drugs which could restore/induce programmes of cell death in a selective way? In considering this end-point of a programmed cell death, which is induced by many drugs in sensitive cells, it has been suggested that there is a cellular hierarchy with respect to the ability of cells to be able to undergo a programme of cell death [73] and that, irrespective of the type of lesion imposed by a drug (whether targeted to membranes or DNA), the cell may only be able to engage apoptosis either if already programmed to do so or if these programmes are initiated. This idea implies that in cells with a high survival potential, new types of drugs may only engage cell death if that survival potential has been attenuated. The modulation of signals which would initiate this process would be fundamental to the promotion of cell loss by apoptosis. Cell death may be one of the adaptive response repertoires open to a cell which has a metabolic imbalance imposed upon it. Unless this programme can be engaged, clever targeting to new biochemistry may still not allow the cellular expression of the desired end point: cell death.

Drugs targeted to the membrane and cell signalling cascades may provide an escape from the current impasse of new drug discovery. The drug industry has been very active in pursuing the types of approaches discussed so far, but little has emerged into the general literature as yet. With a broad approach, accommodating modulation of signals for differentiation, proliferation and apoptosis, the emergence of specific antitumour drugs, rationally designed and targeted, should become a reality.

REFERENCES

1   Rozengurt E: Early signals in the mitogenic response. Science (Washington) 1986 (234):161-166

2   Cantley LC, Auger, KR, Carpenter C, Duckworth B, Graziani A, Kapeller R and Soltoff S: Oncogenes and signal transduction. Cell 1991 (64):281-302

3   Heldin C-H, Betsoltz C, Claesson-Welsh L and Westermark B: Subversion of growth regulatory pathways in malignant transformation. Biochim Biophys Acta 1987 (907):219-244

4   Bishop JM: Molecular themes in oncogenesis. Cell 1991 (64):235-248

5   Rozengurt E: Neuropeptides as cellular growth factors. Eur J Clin Invest 1991 (21):123-134

6   Cuttitta F, Carney DN, Mulshine J, Moody TW, Redorko J, Fischler A and Minna JD: Bombesin-like peptides can function as autocrine growth factors in human small cell lung cancer. Nature (London) 1985 (316):823-826

7   Sinnett-Smith J, Lehman W and Rozengurt E: Bombesin receptor in membranes from Swiss 3T3 cells. Binding characteristics, affinity labelling and modulation by guanine nucleotides. Biochem J 1990 (265):485-493

8   Battey JF, Way JM, Corjay MH, Shapira H, Kusano K, Harkins R, Wu JM, Slattery T, Mann E and Feldman RI: Molecular cloning of the bombesin/GRP receptor from Swiss 3T3 cells. Proc Natl Acad Sci (USA) 1990 (88):395-399

9   Dohlman GH, Thorner J, Caron MG and Lefkowitz RJ: Model systems for the study of seven-transmembrane segment receptors. Ann Rev Biochem 1991 (60):653-688

10 Woll PJ and Rozengurt E: Multiple neuropeptides mobilise calcium in small cell lung cancer: effects of vasopressin, bradykinin, cholecystokinin, galinin and neurotensin. Biochem Biophys Res Commun 1989 (164):66-73

11 Woll PJ and Rozengurt E: A neuropeptide antagonist that inhibits the growth of small cell lung cancer in vitro. Cancer Res 1990 (50):3968-3973

12 Sethi T and Rozengurt E: Multiple neuropeptides mobilise calcium in small cell lung cancer: effects of bradykinin, vasopressin, cholecystokinin, galinin and neurotensin. Cancer Res 1991 (51):3621-3623

13 Yarden Y and Ullrich A: Growth factor receptor tyrosine kinases. Ann Rev Biochem 1988 (57):443-478

14 Jove R and Hanafusa H: Cell transformation by the viral src oncogene. Ann Rev Cell Biol 1987 (3):31-56

15 Presek P and Reuter C: Amiloride inhibits the protein tyrosine kinases associated with the cellular and the transforming src-gene products. Biochem Pharmac 1987 (36):2821-2826

16 Nakano H, Kobayashi E, Takahashi I, Tamaoki T, Kuzuu Y and Iba H: Staurosporine inhibits tyrosine-specific kinase activity of Rous sarcoma virus transforming protein p60. J Antibiot 1987 (40):706-708

17 Kruse CH, Holden KG, Pritchard ML, Feild JA, Rieman DJ, Greig RG and Poste G: Synthesis and evaluation of multisubstrate inhibitors of an oncogene-encoded tyrosine-specific protein kinase. 1. Med Chem 1988 (31):1762-1767

18 Kruse CH, Holden KG, Offen P, Pritchard ML, Feild JA, Rieman DJ, Bender PE, Ferguson B, Greig RG and Poste G: Synthesis and evaluation of multisubstrate inhibitors of an oncogene-encoded tyrosine-specific protein kinase. 2. Med Chem 1988 (263):813-822

19 Fujita-Yamaguchi Y, Sacks DB, McDonald JM, Sahal D and Kathuria S: Effect of basic polycations and proteins on purified insulin receptor. Insulin-independent activation of the receptor tyrosine-specific protein kinase by poly (L-lysine). Biochem J 1989 (263):813-822

20 Geahlen RL and McLaughlin JL: Piceatannol (3,4,3',5'-tetrahydroxy-trans-stilbene) is a naturally occurring protein tyrosine kinase inhibitor. Biochem Biophys Res Commun 1989 (165):241-245

21 Glossman H, Presek P and Eigenbrodt E: Quercetin inhibits tyrosine phosphorylation by the cyclic nucleotide-independent, transforming protein kinase pp60^{src}. Arch Pharmacol 1981 (317):100-103

22 Graziani Y, Erikson E and Erikson RL: The effect of quercetin on the phosphorylation activity of the Rous sarcoma virus transforming gene product in vitro and in vivo. Eur J Biochem 1983 (135):583-589

23 Hanks SK, Quinn AM and Hunter T: The protein kinase family: conserved features and deduced phylogeny of the catalytic domains. Science (Washington) 1988 (241):42-52

24 Akiyama T, Ishida J, Nakagawa S, Ogawara H, Watanabe S, Itoh N, Shibuya M and Fukami Y: Genestein, a specific inhibitor of tyrosine-specific protein kinases. J Biol Chem 1987 (262):5592-5595

25 Geahlen RL, Koonchanok NM, McLaughlin JL and Pratt DE: Inhibition of protein tyrosine kinase activity by flavanoids and related compounds. J Natl Prod 1989 (52):982-986

26 Ogawara H, Akiyama T, Watanabe S, Ito N, Kobori M and Seoda Y: Inhibition of protein tyrosine kinase

activity by synthetic isoflavones and flavones. J Natl Prod 1989 (42):340-343

27 Cunningham B, Threadgill MD. Groundwater PW, Dale I and Hickman JA: Synthesis and biological evaluation of a series of flavones designed as inhibitors of protein tyrosine kinases. 1991 (submitted)

28 Cushman M, Nagarathanmam D, Burg DL and Geahlen RL: Synthesis and protein tyrosine kinase activities of flavanoid analogues. J Med Chem 1991 (34):798-806

29 Geissler JF, Traxler P, Regenass U, Murray BJ, Roesel JL, Meyer T, McGlynn E, Storni A and Lydon NB: Thiazolidine-diones. Biochemical and biological activity of a novel class of tyrosine protein kinase inhibitors. J Biol Chem 1990 (265):22255-22261

30 Imoto M, Umezawa K, Komuro K, Sawa T, Takeuchi T and Umezawa H: Antitumor activity of erbstatin, a tyrosine protein kinase inhibitor. Jpn J Cancer Res 1987 (78):2129-2135

31 Bishop WR, Petrin J, Wang L, Ramesh U and Doll RJ: Inhibition of protein kinase C by the tyrosine kinase inhibitor erbstatin. Biochem Pharmac 1990 (40):2129-2135

32 Toi M, Mukaida H, Wada T, Hirabayashi N, Toge T, Hori H and Umezawa K: Antineoplastic effect of erbstatin on human mammary and esophageal tumors in athymic mice. Eur J Cancer 1990 (26):722-724

33 Levitski A: Tyrphostins - potential antiproliferative agents and novel molecular tools. Biochem Pharmac 1990 (40):913-918

34 Gazit A, Yaish P, Gilon C and Levitski A: Tyrphostins I: synthesis and biological activity of protein tyrosine kinase inhibitors. J Med Chem 1989 (32):2344-2352

35 Posner I, Gazit A, Gilon C and Levitski A: Tyrphostins inhibit the epidermal growth factor receptor-mediated breakdown of phosphoinositides. FEBS Lett 1989 (257):287-291

36 Gazit A, Osherov N, Posner I, Yaish P, Poradosu E, Gilon C and Levitski A: Tyrphostins 2. Heterocyclic and α-substituted benzylidenemalononitrile tyrphostins as potent inhibitors of EGF receptor and ErbB2/neu tyrosine kinases. J Med Chem 1991 (34):1896-1907

37 Slamon DJ, Clark GM, Wong SJ, Levin WJ, Ullrich A and McGuire WJ: Human breast cancer: correlation of relapse and survival with amplification of the HER-2/neu oncogene. Science (Washington) 1987 (235):177-179

38 Faaland A, Mermelstein H, Hayashi J and Laskin JD: Rapid uptake of tyrphostin into A431 human epidermoid cell is followed by delayed inhibition of epidermal growth factor receptor (EGF)-stimulated EGF receptor tyrosine kinase activity. Mol Cell Biol 1991 (11):2697-2703

39 Yoneda T, Lyall RM, Alsina MM, Person PE, Spada AP, Levitski A, Zilberstein A and Mundy GR: The antiproliferative effects of tyrosine kinase inhibitors tyrphostins on a human squamous cell carcinoma in vitro and in nude mice. Cancer Res 1991 (51):4430-4435

40 Shiraishi T, Owada MK, Tatsuka M, Yamashita T, Watanabe K and Kakunaga T: Specific inhibitors of tyrosine-specific protein kinases: properties of 4-hydroxycinnamide derivatives in vitro. Cancer Res 1989 (49):2374-2378

41 Izumi T, Secki Y, Akanuma Y, Takaku F and Kasuga M: Requirement for receptor-intrinsic tyrosine kinase activities during ligand-induced membrane ruffling of KB cells. Essential sites of src-related growth factor receptor kinases. J Biol Chem 1988 (263):10386-10393

42 Kipreos ET and Wang JYJ: Reversible dependence on growth factor interleukin-3 in myeloid cells expressing temperature sensitive v-abl oncogene. Oncogene Res 1988 (2):277-284

43 Koch CA, Anderson D, Moran MF, Ellis C and Pawson T: SH2 and SH3 domains: elements that control interactions of cytoplasmic signalling proteins. Science (Washington) 1991 (252):668-674

44 O'Brien MC, Fukui Y and Hanafusa H: Activation of the proto-oncogene p60-src by point mutations in the SH2 domain. Mol Cell Biol 1990 (10):2855-2862

45 Berridge MJ: Inositol trisphosphate and diacylglycerol: two interacting second messengers. Ann Rev Biochem 1987 (56):159-193

46 Hirata M, Watanabe Y, Ishimatsu T, kebe T, Kimura Y, Yamaguchi K, Ozaki S and Koga T: Synthetic inositol trisphosphate analogs and their effects on phosphatase, kinase and the release of Ca^{2+}. J Biol Chem 1989 (264):20303-20308

47 Safrany ST, Wojcikiewicz RJ, Strupish J, McBain J, Cooke AM, Potter BV and Nahorski SR: Synthetic phosphorothioate-containing analogues of inositol 1,4,5-trisphosphate mobilize intracellular calcium stores and interact differentially with inositol 1,4,5-trisphosphate 5-phosphatase and 3-kinase. Mol Pharmacol 1991 (39):754-761

48 Kemp GJ, Bevington A, Khodja D, Challa A and Russell GG: 32P-labelling anomalies in human erythrocytes. Is there more than one pool of Pi? Biochem J 1989 (264):729-736

49 Powis G, Aksoy IA, Melder DC, Aksoy S, Eichinger H, Fauq AH and Kozikowski AP: D-3-Deoxy-3-substituted myo-inositol analogues as inhibitors of

cell growth. Cancer Chemother Pharmacol 1991 (in press)

50 Gescher A and Dale IL: Protein kinase C - a novel target for rational anticancer drug design? Anticancer Drug Des 1989 (4):93-105

51 O'Brian CA and Ward NE: Biology of the protein kinase C family. Cancer Metastasis Rev 1989 (3):199-214

52 Kikkawa U, Kishimoto A, Nishizuka Y: The protein kinase C family: heterogeneity and its implications. Ann Rev Biochem 1989 (58):31-44

53 Pettit GR, Hartwell JL and Wood HB: Antineoplastic components of marine animals. Nature (London) 1970 (227):962-965

54 Schuchter LM, Esa AH, May WS, Laulis MK, Pettit GR and Hess AD: Successful treatment of murine melanoma with bryostatin 1. Cancer Res 1991 (51):682-687

55 Lilly M, Brown C, Pettit G and Kraft A: Bryostatin 1: a potential antileukemic agent for chronic myelomonocytic leukemia. Leukemia 1991 (5):283-287

56 McCrady CW, Staniswalis J, Pettit GR, Howe C, Grant S: Effect of pharmacological manipulation of protein kinase C by phorbol dibutyrate and bryostatin 1 on the clonogenic response of human granulocyte-macrophage progenitors to recombinant GM-CSF. Br J Haematol 1991 (77):5-15

57 Kraft AS, Smith JB and Berkow RL: Bryostatin, an activator of the calcium phospholipid-dependent protein kinase, blocks phorbol ester-induced differentiation of human promyelocytic leukemia cells HL-60. Proc Natl Acad Sci (USA) 1986 (83):1334-1338

58 Dale IL and Gescher A: Effects of activators of protein kinase C, including bryostatins 1 and 2, on the growth of A549 human lung carcinoma cells. Int J Cancer 1989 (43):158-163

59 Hocevar BA and Fields AP: Selective translocation of β_{II}-protein kinase C to the nucleus of human promyelocytic (HL60) leukemia cells. J Biol Chem 1991 (266):28-33

60 Berdel WE: Membrane-interactive lipids as experimental anticancer drugs. Br J Cancer 1991 (64):208-211

61 Munder PG, Weltzien HU and Modolell M: Lysolecethin analogues: a new class of immunopotentiators. In: Meischer PA (ed) VII International Symposium on Immunopathology. Schwabe Publ, Basel 1977 pp 411-423

62 Bazill W and Dexter TM: Role of endocytosis in the action of ether lipids on WEHI-3B, HL-60, and FDCP-Mix A4 cells. Cancer Res 1990 (50):7505-7512

63 Lazenby CM, Thompson MG and Hickman JA: Elevation of intracellular calcium by the ether lipid SRI62-834. Cancer Res 1990 (50):3327-3330

64 Seewald MJ, Olsen RA, Sehgal I, Melder DC, Modest EJ and Powis G: Inhibition of growth factor-dependent inositol phosphate Ca^{2+} signalling by antitumor ether lipid analogues. Camcer Res 1990 (50):4458-4463

65 Workman P: personal communication

66 Ruoslahti E: Fibronectin and its receptors. Ann Rev Biochem 1988 (57):375-413

67 Barcellos-Hoff MH, Aggeler J, Ram TG and Bissel MJ: Functional differentiation and alveolar morphogenesis of primary mammary epithelial cell cultures on reconstituted basement membrane. Development 1989 (105):223-235

68 Walling JM, Blackmore M, Hickman JA and Townsend KMS: Role of the extracellular matrix on the growth and differentiated phenotype of murine colonic adenocarcinoma cells in vitro. Int J Cancer 1991 (47):776-783

69 La Rocca RV, Stein CA and Myers CE: Suramin: prototype of a new generation of antitumour compounds. Cancer Cells 1990 (2):106-115

70 Waxman S, Rossi GB and Takaku F: The status of differentiation therapy. Serono Symposia. Raven Press, New York 1991

71 Arai K, Lee F, Miyajima A, Miyatake S Arai N and Yokota T: Cytokines: coordinators of immune and inflammatory responses. Ann Rev Biochem 1990 (59):783-836

72 Guy GR, Chua SP, Wong NS, Ng SB and Tan YH: Interleukin 1 and tumor necrosis factor activate common multiple protein kinases in human fibroblasts. J Biol Chem 1991 (266):14343-14352

73 Dive C and Hickman JA: Drug-target interactions: only the first step in the commitment to a programmed cell death? Br J Cancer 1991 (64):192-196

Design of Novel Anti-Endocrine Agents

Michael Jarman

Cancer Research Campaign Laboratories, Drug Development Section, Institute of Cancer Research, Cotswold Road, Belmont, Sutton, Surrey SM2 5NG, United Kingdom

Carcinoma of the breast and prostate are unique among major cancers in that in a high proportion of cases the disease is hormonally controlled and may respond to surgical or therapeutic manipulations designed to ablate hormone synthesis or action [1,2]. Hormonal control is mediated via binding of oestrogenic or androgenic steroids with receptor proteins in the cell, and subsequent interactions of the steroid-receptor complex with DNA. In premenopausal women ovarian aromatase converts the C19 steroids androstenedione and testosterone, synthesised in the adrenals, into oestrone and oestradiol. In postmenopausal women, the source of the much reduced level of circulating oestrogens is aromatization in peripheral tissues [3]. In intact men the testes and to a minor extent the adrenals produce testosterone which is converted into dihydrotestosterone in the prostate gland [4]. Oestradiol and dihydrotestosterone have much higher binding affinities for their respective receptors than oestrone or testosterone and are the principal steroids controlling proliferation in breast and prostatic cancer, respectively.

Since the early 1970s, hormonal antagonism by antiendocrine drugs has been an alternative or supplement to surgical ablation (e.g., oophorectomy, adrenalectomy, orchidectomy) and therapy with natural or synthetic oestrogens. Drugs have been discovered which are variously targeted towards the receptors (antioestrogens and antiandrogens), enzymes in the biosynthetic pathways (Fig.1) leading to oestrogens (aromatase inhibitors), testosterone (17α-hydroxylase-$C_{17,20}$-lyase) or dihydrotestosterone (testosterone 5α-reductase), and feedback control mechanisms (luteinising hormone releasing hormone [LHRH] agonists or antagonists).

Currently-used steroid receptor antagonists and enzyme inhibitors have been markedly less successful in premenopausal women and intact men. Not only is there a high hormone burden to overcome in such patients but hormonal blockade promotes a feedback mechanism to the hypothalamic-pituitary axis stimulating release of luteinising hormone (LH) which acts upon the ovaries or testes to stimulate further steroid synthesis to override the blockade. Since release of LH is in turn controlled by LHRH and occurs only if this is pulsatory, chronic administration of LHRH agonists has been used as a highly successful therapy for prostatic cancer in intact men and a promising alternative to oophorectomy in premenopausal women.

Whilst some of the important antihormonal drugs now used to treat breast and prostatic cancer were not originally designed for this purpose, studies of their mechanism of action and metabolism have guided the design of hopefully more effective congeners. In other cases drugs have been designed *de novo* from rational considerations. Both approaches are exemplified in this selective review which, whilst categorising drugs according to their mode of action, also considers the sometimes controversial matter of the use in sequence or in combination of drugs having different mechanisms of action.

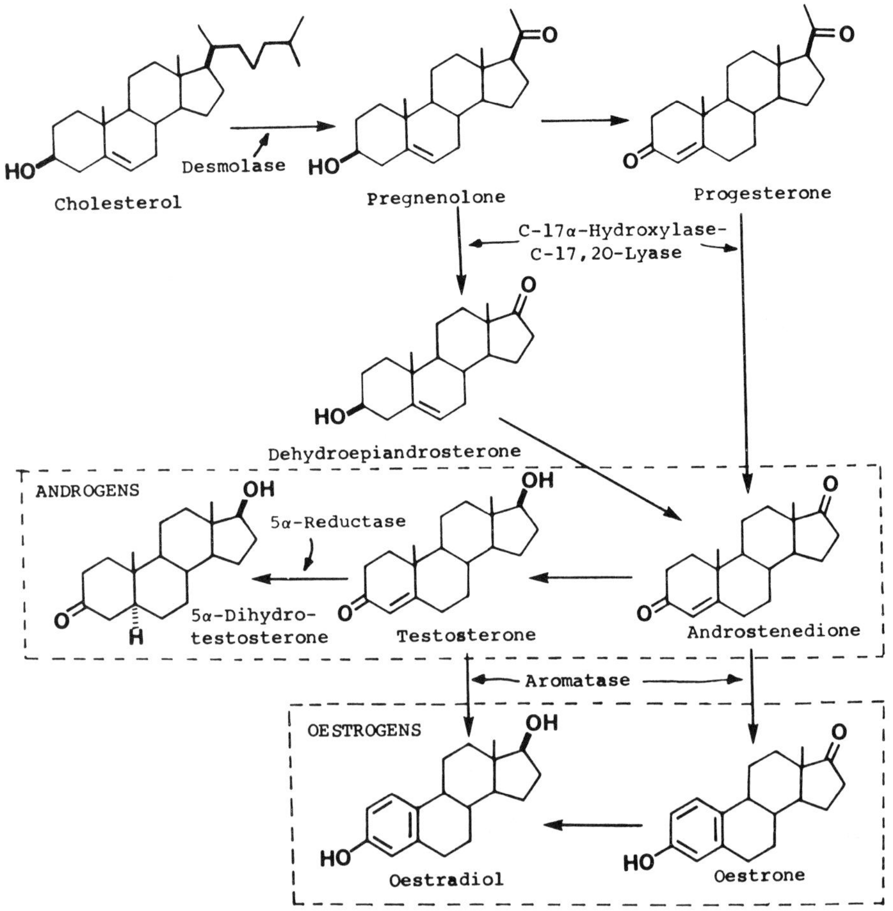

Fig. 1. (Reproduced with permission from ref. 90)

Tamoxifen and the Development of Novel Antioestrogens

It is appropriate to begin the discussion of individual drugs with tamoxifen (ICI, Nolvadex), originally designed as an antifertility agent and first used in the present context in 1971 [5]. In 1988 this accounted for 75% of the market for drugs used to treat breast cancer in the USA [6]. About one-third of patients obtain objective remission (higher in patients selected for receptor status) with the lowest percentage found in premenopausal patients. However, response is temporary, with a median duration of about 14 months [5]. The convenience of oral dosage and minimal toxicity has contributed to the popularity of tamoxifen as a first-line drug therapy in post-menopausal (or oophorectomised premenopausal) patients. Also several trials have given evidence of its efficacy as an adjuvant therapy [7].

It is generally accepted that tamoxifen acts by binding to the oestrogen receptor protein to give a complex which binds to DNA but which lacks the growth-stimulatory action of the oestrogen-receptor complex. However, tamoxifen is not a pure antagonist. Whereas it counteracts oestrogen-stimulated uterine growth in immature rats given oestradiol, when administered without oestrogen it *stimulates* uterine growth. This partial agonist action may contribute to the emergence of resistance to tamoxifen in patients still responsive to aromatase inhibitors (see later) but partial agonism could also prevent the onset of osteoporosis in post-menopausal women [8].

This controversy regarding the disadvantages or otherwise of the partial agonist action has stimulated the search for compounds having reduced agonist or even pure antagonist activity. Another important issue is potency. Tamoxifen has a relatively modest affinity for the oestrogen receptor, only about 1% of that of oestradiol (relative binding affinity, RBA = 1

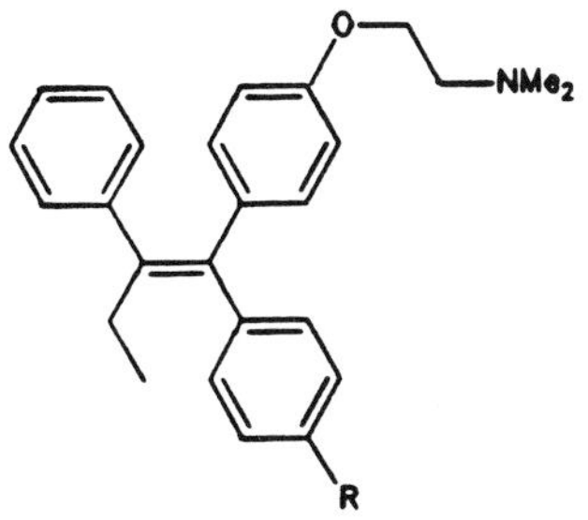

(trans) tamoxifen: R=H
4−hydroxytamoxifen: R=OH

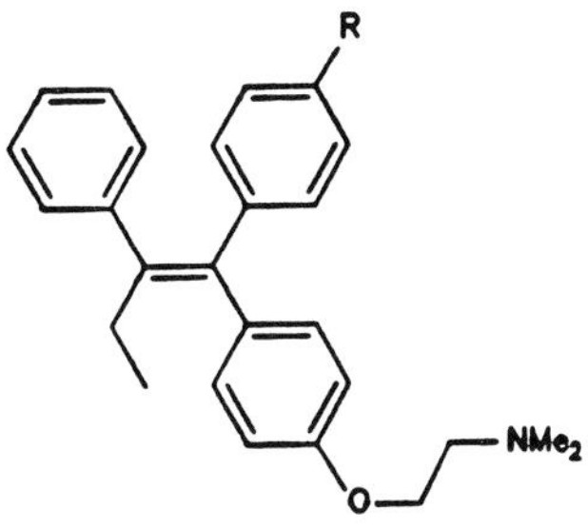

(cis) tamoxifen: R=H
4−hydroxytamoxifen: R=OH

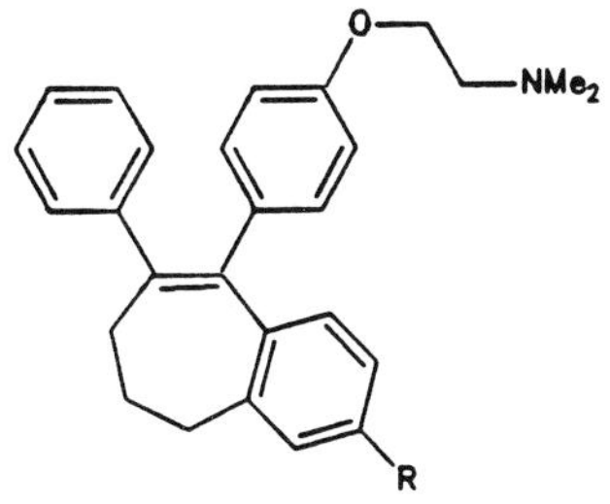

fixed ring (trans) analogues

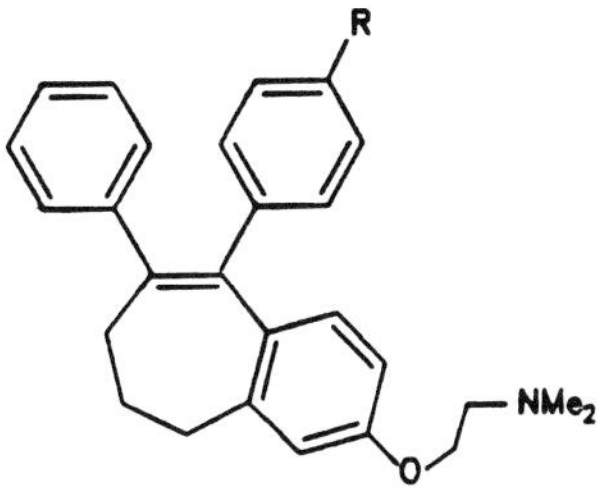

fixed ring (cis) analogues

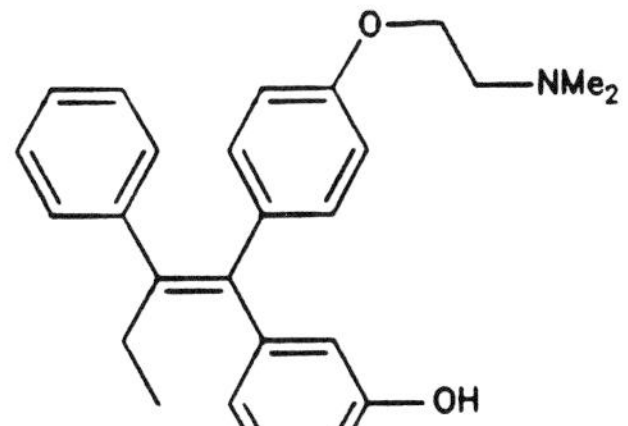

droloxifene

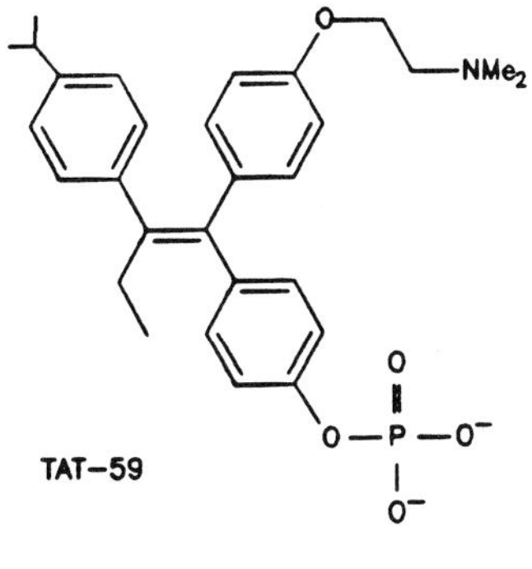

TAT−59

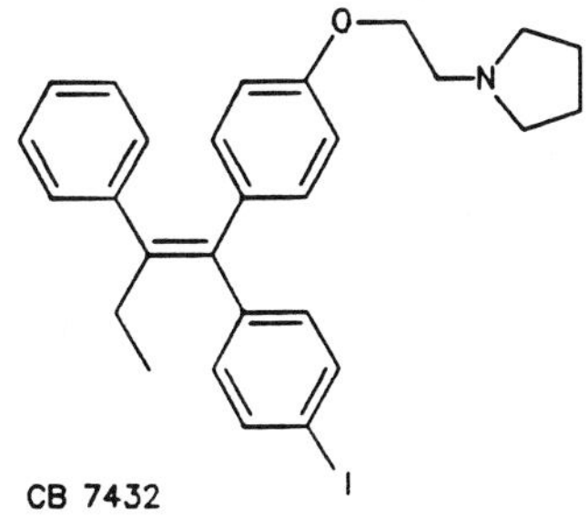

CB 7432

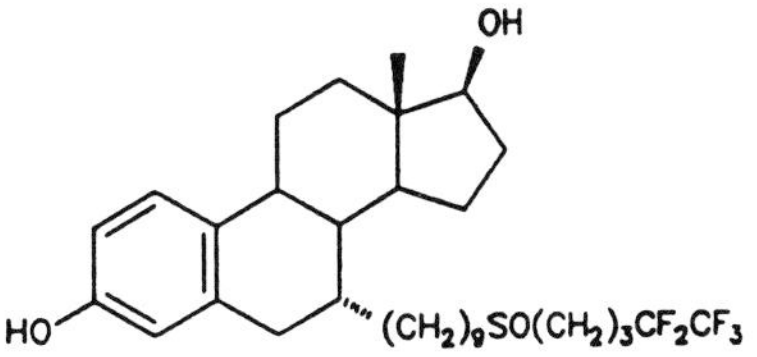

ICI 182 780

on a scale where oestradiol = 100). Actions on cell signalling pathways are also relevant, particularly calmodulin. The oestrogen receptor is a phosphoprotein. A phosphorylation-dephosphorylation cycle is implicated in its biological actions and phosphorylation on tyrosine is stimulated by calmodulin [9]. It has been proposed that the reported inhibition of calmodulin-dependent phosphodiesterase by tamoxifen may be relevant to the drug's antioestrogenic action [10].

Consideration of the metabolites of tamoxifen [5] is important since these can vary both in their RBA value, in the balance between oestrogenicity and antioestrogenicity, and in pharmacokinetic properties. In patients' plasma, N-desmethyltamoxifen is the major metabolite, but is similar in all these properties to tamoxifen. 4-Hydroxytamoxifen is a minor metabolite in terms of plasma concentration but because of its high RBA value (equal to oestradiol) could contribute importantly to tamoxifen's therapeutic effects. It is readily converted at physiological pH into the cis-isomer [11]. Since cis-tamoxifen is an oestrogen it seemed possible that cis-4-hydroxytamoxifen might be also. This concern was allayed in an ingenious way by making analogues which could not interconvert. "Fixed-ring" analogues of both trans and cis 4-hydroxytamoxifen (and of tamoxifen itself) were synthesised and shown to antagonise growth stimulation by oestradiol of MCF-7 cells or rat uterus growth, though the cis isomer was the less potent [12]. The dimethylaminoethyl side-chain is important for antagonist activity. Allowed variations on this side-chain are other basic substituents or an appropriately located hydroxyl or ester function [13].

Based on the established need for an appropriate side-chain and the high binding affinity conferred by the 4-hydroxyl substituent, a number of analogues of tamoxifen have been synthesised and are in various stages of clinical or preclinical development. Relocation of the hydroxyl group to the 3-position (droloxifene) [14], conversion of the 4-hydroxy derivative to a modified phosphate ester (TAT-59) [15] and replacement of 4-hydroxyl by another appropriate substituent (the iodinated pyrrolidino derivative CB7432 [16]) are all variations which have produced compounds retaining substantially higher RBA values than tamoxifen with evidence for reduced oestrogenicity. Also under clinical trial is another variant of tamoxifen in which the ethyl group is replaced by chloroethyl to give a compound (toremifene) with the same RBA value but improved antioestrogenic profile in the rat [17].

An alternative approach has been the development of steroidal oestrogen receptor antagonists. 7-Substituted oestradiol derivatives, of which the most potent reported is ICI 182, 780, [18] are not only devoid of uterotrophic activity in rats, but achieve their antiuterotrophic effects without affecting gonadotrophin secretion from the pituitary in intact rats. Translated into the clinical setting such compounds (unlike tamoxifen) should not block central negative oestrogen feedback and hence should not stimulate oestrogen production in the premenopausal patient. The growing knowledge of the structure of the oestrogen receptor and the biological mechanisms whereby tamoxifen exerts its antioestrogenic effects will undoubtedly help in the design of novel oestrogen antagonists. The oestrogen receptor gene has now been sequenced, cloned and expressed [19] and the binding site with oestrogen and with DNA probed by the use of a chemically reactive oestrogen and antioestrogen [20]. A breakthrough in our understanding of the way in which tamoxifen exerts its cytostatic effects has come from the work of Lippman and coworkers who described an 8-17 fold enhancement of TGF-ß secretion from MCF-7 cells treated with tamoxifen or 4-hydroxytamoxifen [21]. They proposed that TGF-ß acts as a negative autocrine growth factor. They also found inhibition of an oestrogen receptor-negative cell line cocultured with MCF-7 indicating that tamoxifen could be effective in a heterogeneous population by a paracrine growth factor effect. Induction of TGF-ß by tamoxifen may also be an important mechanism in the adjuvant setting [8]. Conversely, however, antioestrogen-irreversible growth *stimulation* of MCF-7 cells cocultured with an excess of a hormone-independent cell line MDA-MB-231 shows that the paracrine effect can operate adversely [22]. Finally, important insights into the mechanism of acquired resistance to tamoxifen therapy which is an inevitable clinical outcome are emerging from the experimental observation that xenografted MCF-7 human breast cancer cells in nude mice escape from suppression after 3-4 months of therapy with the drug [23].

Inhibitors of Aromatase

Whereas antioestrogens act by inhibiting the *action* of oestrogens, aromatase inhibitors act by blocking their synthesis. Until recently the only aromatase inhibitor to be widely and successfully used in the clinic was aminoglutethimide (Ciba-Geigy, Orimeten) [24]. Originally developed as an antiepileptic drug, its withdrawal because it caused adrenal insufficiency led to its reintroduction in the early

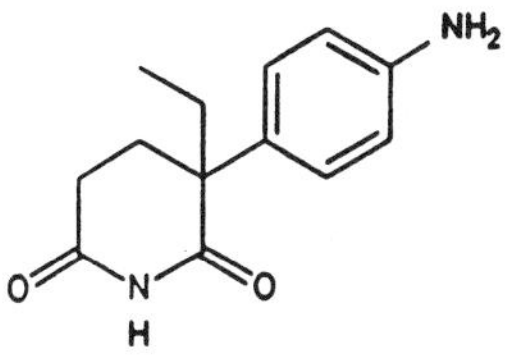

aminoglutethimide

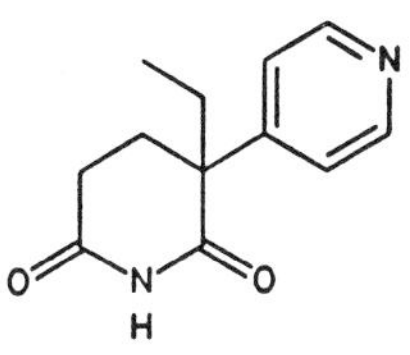

rogletimide

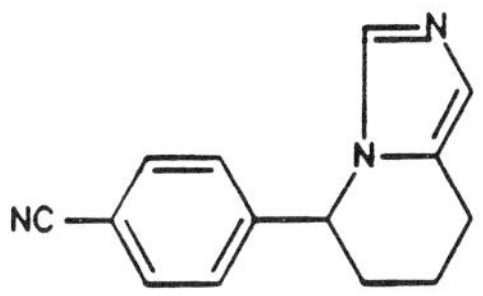

CGS 16949A

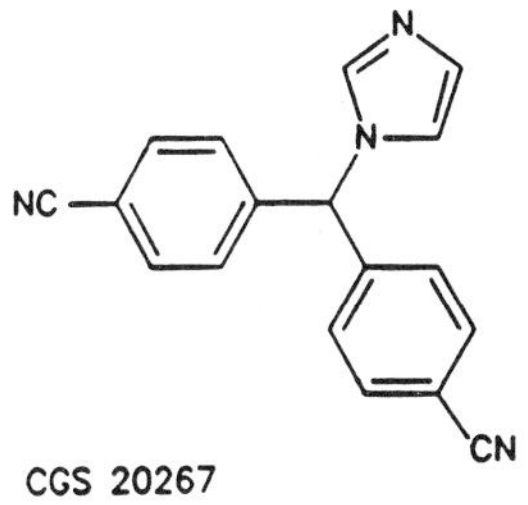

CGS 20267

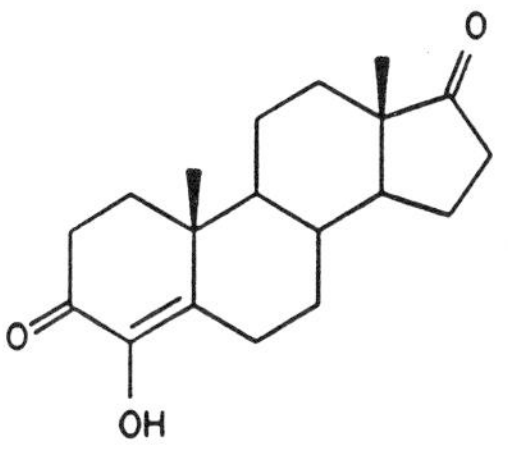

CPG 32349

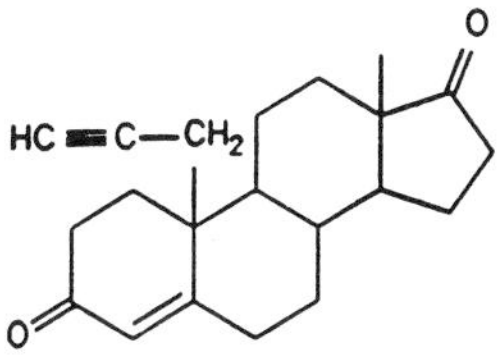

MDL 18962

1970s as an antihormonal agent to treat breast cancer and the subsequent discovery that its principal site of action in this context was inhibition of aromatase [25].

Response rates and duration of response on aminoglutethimide in postmenopausal patients are very similar to those with tamoxifen. However, patients who relapse on tamoxifen may respond to aminoglutethimide as second-line therapy [26]. This complementarity implies different mechanisms of escape from hormonal response for the two agents.

Aminoglutethimide is not an ideal drug. Side effects, particularly sedation, can be troublesome. It is not a selective aromatase inhibitor. Several other steroidogenic pathways are inhibited and corticosteroids are depleted, necessitating replacement therapy. It can cause haematologic toxicity, probably through formation of a toxic hydroxylamine metabolite [27]. It is an inducer of hepatic metabolism, and the failure of the combination of tamoxifen and aminoglutethimide to elicit response rates superior to either drug alone has been attributed to the enhanced rate of clearance of tamoxifen induced by aminoglutethimide [28]. These drawbacks have prompted the search in recent years for a selective aromatase inhibitor, hopefully of greater potency, which lacks the other adverse features of aminoglutethimide.

The non-steroidal inhibitors of aromatase are thought to act via a reversible reaction of a basic residue with the haem moiety which is present in aromatase and other oxidative enzymes of the cytochrome P-450 type [29]. Inhibitors possessing imidazole, triazole, pyridine and pyrimidine substituents have been exemplified [6]. The one most closely related to aminoglutethimide which has been clinically evaluated is the pyridine analogue (U.S. Bioscience, rogletimide) [30], of only comparable potency but a selective aromatase inhibitor [31]. Selective inhibitors of much greater potency are now under trial. For example CGS 16949A (Ciba-Geigy) is therapeutically effective at 1-2 mg b.d. but is not entirely selective, suppressing aldosterone at these dose levels [32]. However, this problem appears to have been overcome in the even more potent CGS 20267 [33].

The lack of obvious structural resemblance between these non-steroidal inhibitors and the substrates for aromatase raises the question of their mechanisms of action. Recently, molecular modelling studies, now playing an increasing role in drug discovery, have envisaged these inhibitors as mimics of the steroidal substrates for aromatase. Their basic residue is orientated in the general direction which the C-19 methyl group occupies. The latter is oxidised by a 3-step process (Scheme 1) involving an oxygenating species coordinated to a haem iron residue [34]. In the case of rogletimide the pyridine

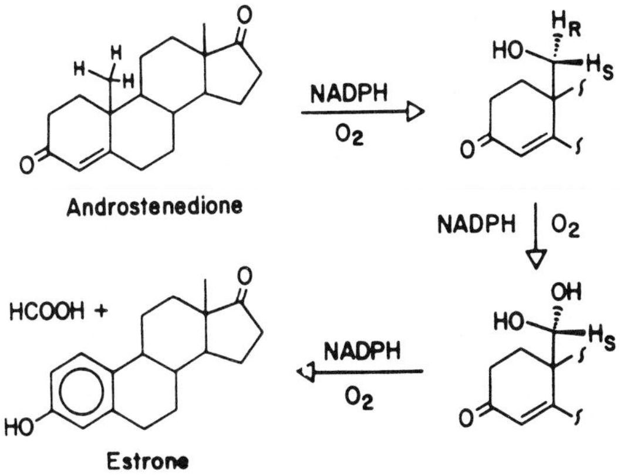

Androstenedione

Estrone

Scheme 1. (Reproduced with permission from ref. 34)

nitrogen would coordinate to the haem iron and the glutarimide ring would mimic ring A of the steroid, one of its carbonyl functions overlapping the position which would be occupied by the 3-keto function [35]; in the CGS compounds the imidazole nitrogen and the polar cyano group would respectively perform these roles [36]. Such models can rationalise known structure-activity relationships and also have predictive value [35].

Steroidal inhibitors of aromatase have also been developed. Potential problems with these include oral effectiveness and alternative steroid-like actions of the drug and its metabolites. Nevertheless, 4-hydroxyandrostenedione (Ciba-Geigy, CGP 32349), a rationally developed [37] analogue of the natural substrate androstenedione, and a potent and selective aromatase inhibitor, has proved to suppress oestradiol effectively in both oral and parenteral dosage [38]. It appears to be an irreversible inhibitor of aromatase by an unknown mechanism. Other potent irreversible steroidal aromatase inhibitors have been designed. The general principle is to introduce a suitable substituent in place of the C-19 methyl group of the natural substrate which can be oxidised by aromatase but produces a grouping reactive towards amino acids in the binding site. The propynyl derivative MDL 18962 is a prototype example of an aromatase inhibitor designed using this approach [39].

A controversy in the field of aromatase inhibitors concerns the question of whether the new generation of inhibitors will necessarily give higher response rates in the clinic than aminoglutethimide. Using double labelling techniques which measure directly the efficiency with which drugs inhibit the aromatisation of androstenedione in humans, aminoglutethimide was reported to be at least 95% inhibitory at a dose of 1 g daily [25] whereas the much more potent inhibitor CGS 16949A was also highly inhibitory (93%) at 2 mg b.d. [40]. However, it is well established that plasma levels of oestrogen are not depressed to this degree during therapy: for example, in typical studies levels of oestradiol and oestrone fell to only 45-65% of pretreatment values during therapy [24] with aminoglutethimide and to 67% and 28% on CGS 16949A [41]. The implication is that there are other sources of oestrogen besides aromatase-mediated reactions. One possibility is the action of oestrone sulphatase on the circulating conjugate oestrone sulphate which can act as a depot form for oestrone [42]. Inhibitors of this enzyme may therefore need to be developed for use in conjunction with aromatase inhibitors. Despite doubts as to whether complete oestrogen ablation is attainable using aromatase inhibitors it may be hoped that a highly potent inhibitor might have utility in premenopausal patients as well as improving response rates postmenopausally.

Luteinising Hormone Releasing Hormone (LHRH) Analogues

The controlled biosynthesis of steroids in the ovaries and testes depends upon the pulsatile release of the decapeptide LHRH from the hypothalamus. Continuous administration of large doses of LHRH or an analogue (agonist) on the other hand leads, by the third week of treatment, to a 75% suppression of plasma testosterone levels [43]. Although some promise has been shown in the use of LHRH agonists against breast cancer in premenopausal women [44], their major application has been in the treatment of advanced prostatic cancer as an alternative to high-dose oestrogen therapy or orchidectomy [45]. The design of LHRH agonists has recently been extensively reviewed [44]. Very briefly, the aim has been to produce a stabler, more potent analogue of natural LHRH by judicious replacement of residues in the decapeptide by amino acids of unnatural (D) configuration and by synthetic lipophilic amino acids. The present account will concentrate on the important issue of complementarity between LHRH analogues and drugs having other mechanisms of action in the treatment of advanced prostatic cancer.

Many clinical trials have attested to the success of LHRH agonists in achieving castrate levels of testosterone and dihydrotestosterone and responses equivalent to those achieved with orchidectomy [46]. The painful "tumour flare" caused by an initial rise in testosterone levels during the first few days of therapy can, in principle, be overcome by the use of LHRH *antagonists* but their development has been slow, in part due to problems with histamine release [47].

An LHRH agonist can only ablate *testicular* androgen synthesis which accounts for approximately 95% of the total, the remainder occurring in the adrenals. In practice, androgen levels after LHRH agonist treatment can be somewhat higher than expected from these figures; in one study testosterone was suppressed to 25% and dihydrostestosterone to 10% of pretreatment levels by treatment for 3 months with the LHRH agonist Zoladex (ICI) [48]. This concern over residual androgen synthesis has led to the concept of total androgen ablation by combining an LHRH agonist (or castration) with an antiandrogen to blockade the action of residual androgen at the level of the androgen receptor [49]. For example, in a study of patients who relapsed on orchidectomy, oestrogen therapy or LHRH agonist alone, treatment with LHRH agonist combined with the antiandrogen flutamide gave a further objective response in 34.5% of patients [50]. Blockade of adrenal androgen biosynthesis by inhibitors of 17α-hydroxylase/$C_{17,20}$-lyase is an alternative strategy. The role of drugs having these alternative modes of action is considered in the following sections. Two recent reports indicate an advantage in giving the combined treatment of an antiandrogen and LHRH analogue or castration to achieve total androgen ablation. A median survival advantage of 41.2 compared with 24 months was reported in a trial comparing the combination with recent results of trials using monotherapy only [51]. In a randomised double blind trial comparing Leuprolide (Abbot) + flutamide with Leuprolide alone the increased median survival was 35 vs 27.9 months accompanied by longer progression-free survival [52]. However, it is fair to say that other trials have produced results which are much less supportive of the advantages of the combined treatment [53,54].

Flutamide and the Development of Novel Antiandrogens

Two antiandrogens established in clinical use are the steroidal drug cyproterone acetate and the non-steroidal flutamide (Schering) [55]. Neither was designed for the present application. Cyproterone acetate was developed as an orally active progestogen for use as an abortificient [56]. Here attention is confined to flutamide. This was developed as a bacteriostatic agent but subsequently shown to be a pure antiandrogen. Much work on rational analogue design has been carried out. Flutamide is used following orchidectomy, or in conjunction with an LHRH agonist. This is because in intact patients antagonism of androgen at the hypothalamic-pituitary level leads to a compensatory increase in circulating gonadotrophins and consequently of testosterone synthesis in the testes, resulting in escape from androgen suppression [57].

The goal in the development of a successor to flutamide has been a drug effective against androgen-dependent disease without causing a compensatory rise in hormonal levels. A successful approach has developed from an understanding of the role of hydroxyflutamide. This is a major metabolite of flutamide in men [58], having 40-fold flutamide's binding of affinity to the androgen receptor *in vitro*. It is therefore believed to be essentially responsible for the *in vivo* effects of flutamide. Although apparently unrelated in structure to dihydrotestosterone, flutamide was noted from molecular models to resemble it in having a largely flat structure [59]. Modelling of hydroxyflutamide ascribed its greater binding affinity to its dominant conformation in which the amide NH bond eclipsed the hydroxyl function [60]. Of similar binding affinity to hydroxyflutamide is a related antiandrogen Anandron (Roussel Uclef) which is a conformationally fixed equivalent of hydroxyflutamide [61]. A recent elaboration on the 4-hydroxyflutamide structure in which there is a further intramolecular interaction of the hydroxyl group is ICI 176,334 [60]. In this compound the goal of an antiandrogen with effects confined to the accessory sex organs appears to have been largely achieved, at least experimentally. In intact rats the compound elevated testosterone levels by only 2-fold (4-fold for flutamide) and LHRH levels not at all (7-fold for flutamide). It appears that ICI 176,334 does not penetrate androgen receptor-containing neurons in the hypothalamus and thus does not block negative feedback of endogenous androgens [62]. An orally active steroidal androgen receptor antagonist which

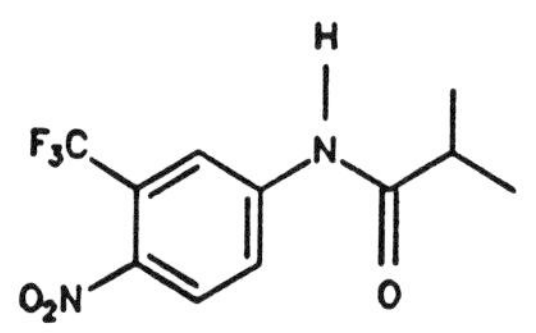

flutamide

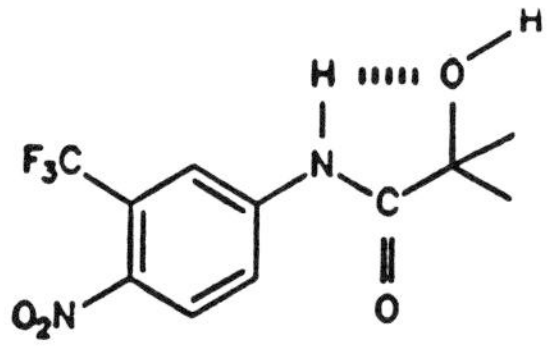

hydroxyflutamide

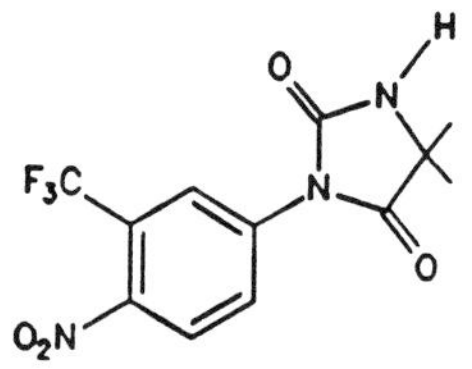

anandron

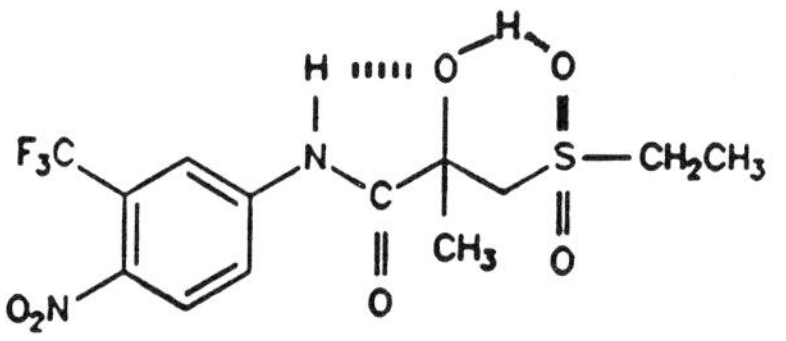

ICI 176 334

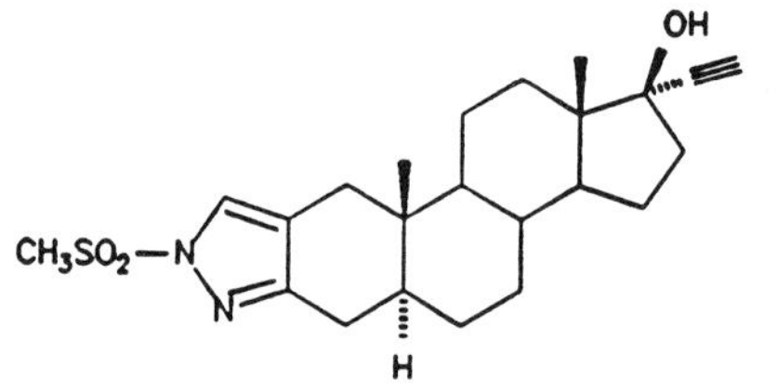

WIN 49596

also appears to possess these desirable properties is WIN 49596 (Sterling Winthrop) [63]; this is unique among steroidal antiandrogens in possessing no demonstrable hormone agonist activity.

Inhibitors of 17α-Hydroxylase/C$_{17,20}$-Lyase

The biosynthesis of dehydroepiandrosterone and androstenedione, immediate precursors of testosterone, from pregnenolone and progesterone, respectively, occurs by a 2-step pathway with their 17α-hydroxy derivatives as intermediates [64]. As with flutamide, inhibitors of this hydroxylase/lyase pathway are primarily envisaged as suppressing residual androgen synthesis in the adrenals following orchidectomy, or for use in conjunction with LHRH analogues. An agent having this locus of action which has been quite extensively evaluated clinically is ketoconazole (Janssen) [65]. Originally introduced for use as an antifungal agent, observation of gynaecomastia in some men given the drug led to the discovery that it depleted plasma testosterone levels and hence to its use in the present context. Aminoglutethimide, for which successful use against prostatic cancer has been reported, was originally thought to act by ablating steroidal androgens through inhibiting cholesterol side-chain cleavage but is now thought to act by other mechanisms [66]. In an open multicentre trial of 400 patients with metastatic prostate cancer the objective response rate for previously untreated patients was 71% and 34% for those who previously relapsed on hormonal treatment [28]. Suppression of cortisol is a potential drawback of hydroxylase/lyase inhibitors, since 17α-hydroxyprogesterone is its immediate precursor, but was not found in this study. There have been both experimental and clinical studies which attest to the potential value of combining ketoconazole with an

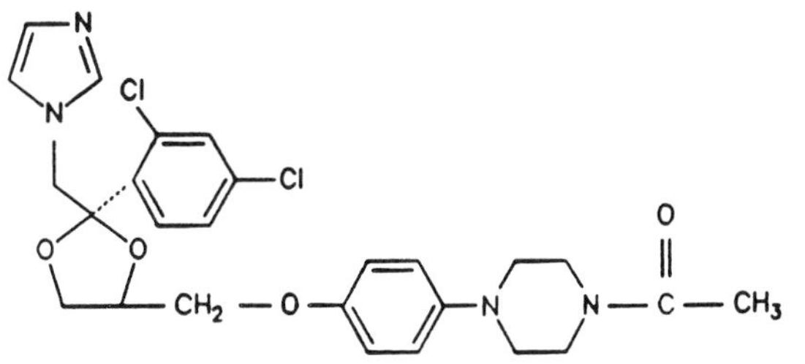

ketoconazole

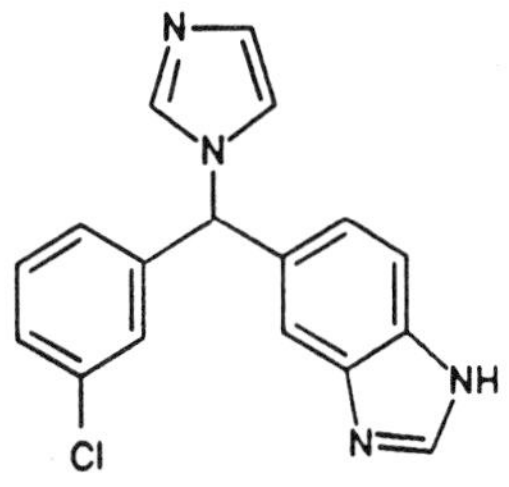

R 75251

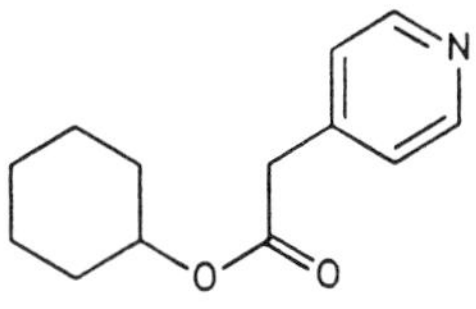

cyclohexyl 4−pyridylacetate

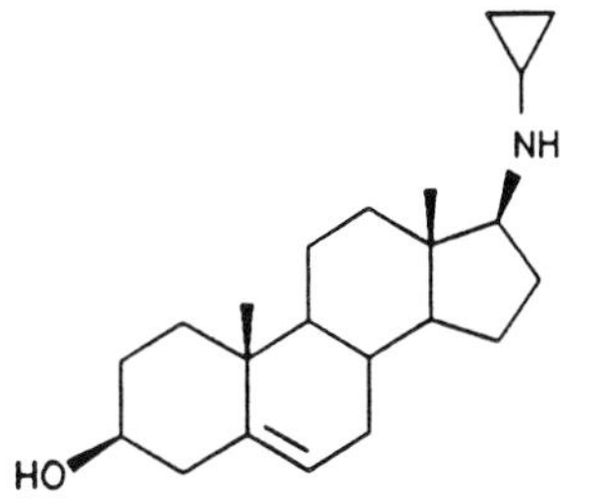

MDL 27301

LHRH analogue or orchidectomy. In the rat, ketoconazole combined with leuprolide gave a greater suppression of testosterone than either agent given alone [67]. The ability of ketoconazole to suppress testicular as well as adrenal androgen biosynthesis is attested by the aforementioned clinical responses seen in intact patients. Also there was a fall in androstenedione, dehydroepiandrosterone and testosterone levels (though not cortisol) in patients treated with ketoconazole (600 mg/day) prior to orchidectomy in whom adrenals were suppressed with dexamethazone, and marked falls in hydroxylase/lyase activity in testes examined after orchidectomy [68].

Despite some clinical successes, gastrointestinal and other toxicities and the inconvenience of the 3 x daily dosage necessitated by the short half-life of ketoconazole have prompted its withdrawal and the search for improved inhibitors. An imidazole derivative which proved more potent than ketoconazole in suppressing testosterone levels in male volunteers to castrate range is R 75251 (Janssen) [69]. A particularly powerful aromatase inhibitor (IC_{50} = 2.9 nM) and a reasonably effective (submicromolar) inhibitor of hydroxylase/lyase, R 75251 was, despite its testosterone inhibition, much less effective

than ketoconazole in suppressing the adrenal androgens dehydroepiandrosterone and androstenedione. Hence there is doubt that hydroxylase/lyase inhibition is its principal mode of action in this context and indeed preliminary evidence for its clinical utility in hormone *refractory* cancer has been reported [70].

Development of other inhibitors is at an experimental stage. The serendipitous discovery that certain esters of 4-pyridylacetic acid (e.g., cyclohexyl 4-pyridylacetate) originally designed as inhibitors of aromatase also inhibited hydroxylase/lyase [71] was the basis of an analogue programme which has, in part, been guided by molecular modelling. As with aromatase, the pyridine nitrogen atom is envisaged as coordinating with haem iron, this time in the region of the C_{17}-C_{20} bond, which places the hydrophobic portion of the inhibitor in the general region occupied by that of the steroidal ring B [72]. As with aromatase the sequence, though not the 3-dimensional structure of human hydroxylase/lyase, is known [73]. Based on limited sequence homology with the cytochrome P-450_{cam}, the only cytochrome P-450 enzyme where the full structure is known [74], a 3-dimensional model of hydroxylase/lyase has been constructed which could prove helpful in guiding the design of an improved inhibitor [75].

As with aromatase, consideration of the mechanism of the biochemical pathway mediated by hydroxylase/lyase has guided the rational design of a mechanism-based irreversible steroidal inhibitor, MDL 27301 (Merrell Dow) [76]. This contains a substituent (cyclopropylamino) at the position equivalent to that occupied by the 2-carbon side-chain which is cleaved from the natural substrate pregnenolone. Based on the proposed mechanism [77] for oxidative cleavage of the C_{17}-C_{20} bond, oxidation at nitrogen (probably by Fe^{III}-OOH) followed by opening of the cyclopropyl ring gives a ß-iminium radical which can form a covalent bond with the enzyme resulting in powerful irreversible inhibition ($K_i$app = 90 nM).

Inhibitors of Testosterone 5α-Reductase

The identification of dihydrotestosterone as the principal active androgen in the prostate [78] and its formation in that organ by enzymatic reduction of testosterone makes inhibition of testosterone 5α-reductase an attractive target for the treatment of prostatic cancer. A further attraction is that ablation of dihydrotestosterone in the prostate does not interfere with testosterone production and normal testicular function.

In contrast with other classes of antiendocrine drug, serendipity has played little part in the discovery of 5α-reductase inhibitors. Rather, their design has been mechanism- based, on the hypothesis that enzymatic reduction of the 4-ene-3-one residue in testosterone involves transfer of hydrogen from the reduced cofactor NADPH to the 5α-position of the steroid resulting in a 3-enol transition state intermediate (Scheme 2). Petrow et al. designed irreversible inhibitors (e.g. 6-methyleneprogesterone) based on the idea that the 6-methylene substituent might react with nucleophilic sites on the enzyme by an analogous mechanism [79]. More recently, X-ray crystal analysis of such 6-methylene substituted steroids and close structural analogues in relation to their inhibitory activities has led to the conclusion, potentially helpful in inhibitor design, that the 5α-reductase enzyme possesses a narrow hydrophobic pocket which accommodates the C-6 substituent [80]. More potent (K_i values ca. 10^{-8}M), reversible competitive inhibitors are azasteroids exemplified by 4-MA (Merck, Sharp and Dohme), which were envisaged as mimics of the transition state [81]. 4-MA was active against a prostatic tumour model in the Noble rat [82], but has potentially a dual mechanism of action since it also binds to the androgen receptor [81]. The structurally related finasteride (Merck, Sharp and Dohme, MK 906) which, unlike 4-MA, does not bind to the androgen receptor has received a clinical trial on stage D prostatic cancer with results which warrant its further study [83]. In volunteers it produced a 65% decrease in plasma levels of dihydrotestosterone on day 1 at a dose of only 1 mg/day [84].

In principle, competitive inhibitors of 5α-reductase such as the azasteroids could induce a build-up of testosterone behind the blockade, eventually overcoming the inhibitory effect [85]. This potential drawback can be overcome by taking advantage of certain features of the reductive process. Thus, 5α-reduction is an ordered sequential mechanism in which the reduced cofactor NADPH binds first, followed by testosterone, the order

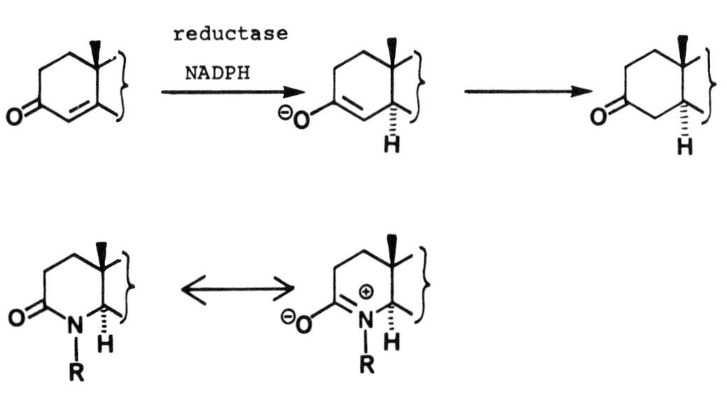

Scheme 2.
(Reproduced with permission from ref. 90)

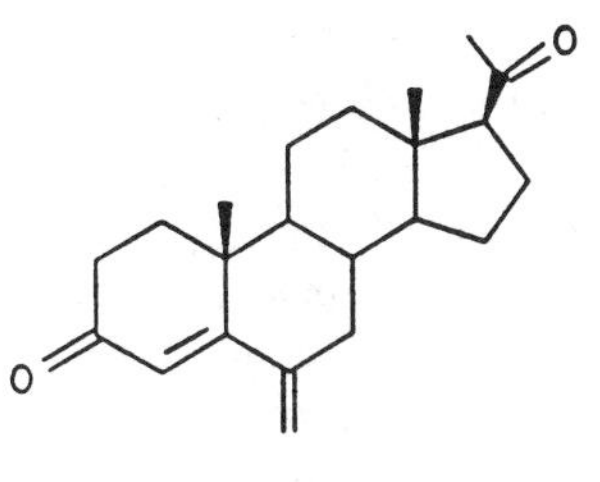

6-methyleneprogesterone

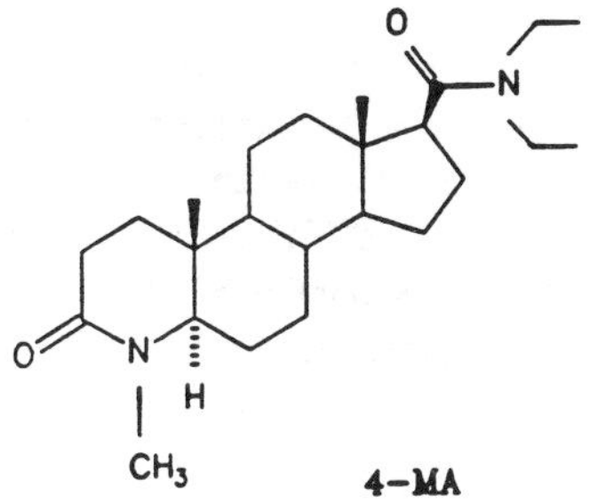

4-MA

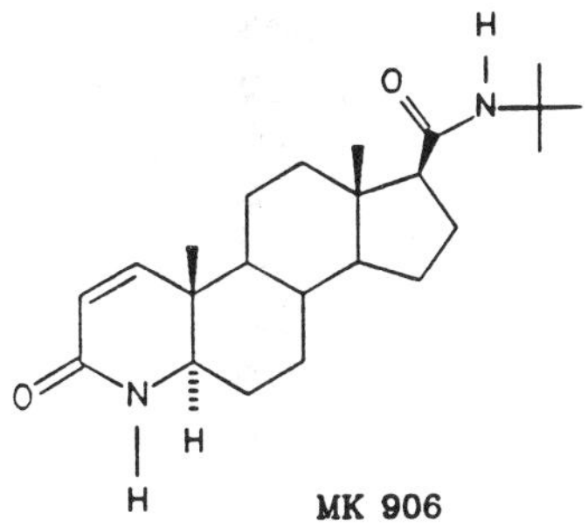

MK 906

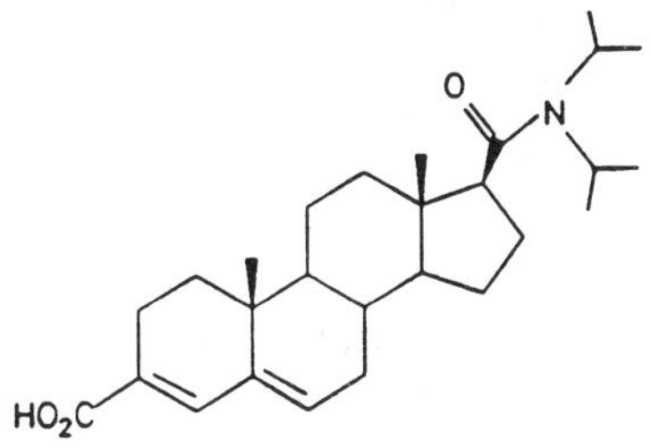

steroidal acrylate

of release of the products being dihydrotestosterone followed by NADP+ [86]. This mechanism has been exploited in the design of novel steroid acrylates, transition state analogues which powerfully inhibit the 5α-reductase (Kii 11 ± 1 nM) by forming a ternary complex with the enzyme and NADP+ [87]. A key feature of steroidal acrylates is their possession of an ionizable carboxyl function: the anion interacting with the positive charge on the oxidised form of the cofactor. The inhibition is uncompetitive with respect to testosterone and should not therefore be overcome by its accumulation.

As with the other target enzymes described here, the 5α-reductase has been cloned and expressed in simian COS cells enabling the properties of enzyme from rat and human to be compared in detail [88]. Since the sequence homology between the 2 species was only 60%, species differences in inhibitory potency for a given inhibitor are to be expected and indeed were reported from a previous study [89] comparing the potency of various azasteroids as inhibitors of enzyme preparations from dog, human and rat prostate. What was unexpected, not having been seen in that study, was the disparate inhibitory potencies of 4-MA (Ki = 3-5 nM) and finasteride (Ki = 340-620 nM) towards the cloned human enzyme [88], a difference

particularly puzzling in view of the potency of finasteride in depressing dihydrotestosterone in the volunteer study [84]. The reason for these discrepancies remains to be clarified.

Conclusions

It will be seen that considerable advances have been made in the design of potential drugs having increased affinity and selectivity for the various target enzymes and receptors considered here. Actual or potential drawbacks of existing agents have been identified and circumvented. Taking the categories in turn, the availability of a pure antioestrogen for clinical evaluation will enable the advantages or otherwise of such an agent over tamoxifen to be established. The current generation of aromatase inhibitors includes examples of such potency and selectivity that the clinical potential of inhibitors of this target can be definitively assessed. This is not the case for inhibitors of the other cytochrome P-450 enzyme target hydroxylase/lyase. Here the scope for improvements, possibly exploiting a knowledge of enzyme structure, is considerable. The role of inhibitors of this enzyme, and of antiandrogens, in relation to the

LHRH analogues remains a controversial question perhaps best answered by the development of new agents much improved on ketoconazole and flutamide. Regarding the latter, the development of compounds which, at least experimentally, can inhibit androgen receptor binding without markedly elevating testosterone levels is a notable advance. However, as with pure antioestrogens with effects confined to the accessory sex organs, it remains to be seen whether this experimental achievement can be translated into clinical practice. Finally, although primarily designed for the treatment of benign prostatic hypertrophy, inhibitors of testosterone 5α-reductase have undoubted potential in the treatment of prostatic cancer, particularly now that the potential problem of elevated testosterone levels overcoming the enzyme blockade has been circumvented.

One may question whether all these antiendocrine therapies are doomed to remain palliative rather than curative treatments for advanced disease, owing to the heterogeneity of the target cell populations. At least the new treatments should help to provide a definitive answer to this question.

REFERENCES

1   Jensen EV: Hormone dependency of breast cancer. Cancer 1981 (47):2319-2326

2   Grayhack JT, Keeler TC and Kozlowski MD: Carcinoma of the prostate. Hormonal therapy. Cancer 1987 (60):589-601

3   Brodie AMH, Banks PK, Inkster SE et al: Aromatase and other inhibitors in breast and prostatic cancer. J Steroid Biochem Molec Biol 1990 (37):1043-1048

4   Cunha GR, Donjacour AA, Cooke PS et al: The endocrinology and developmental biology of the prostate. Endocrine Reviews 1987 (8):338-361

5   Furr BJ and Jordan VC: The pharmacology and clinical uses of tamoxifen. Pharmac Ther 1984 (25):127-205

6   Cole PA and Robinson CH: Mechanism and inhibition of cytochrome P-450 aromatase. J Med Chem 1990 (33):2933-2942

7   Smith I: Adjuvant tamoxifen for early breast cancer. Br J Cancer 1988 (57):527-528

8   Fentiman IS: Breast cancer prevention with tamoxifen. Eur J Cancer 1990 (26):655-656

9   Migliaccio A, Rotondi A and Auricchio F: Calmodulin-stimulated phosphorylation of 17ß-estradiol receptor in tyrosine. Proc Natl Acad Sci USA 1984 (81):5921-5925

10   Fanidi A, Courion-Guichardaz C, Fayard J-M et al: Inhibition of Ca^{2+}-calmodulin dependent phosphodiesterase in quail oviduct. Endocrinology 1989 (125):1187-1193

11   Katzenellenbogen JA, Carlson KE and Katzenellenbogen BS: Facile geometrical isomerization of phenolic non-steroidal estrogens and antiestrogens: limitations to the interpretation of experiments characterizing the activity of individual isomers. J Steroid Biochem 1985 (22):589-596

12   McCague R, Leclercq G and Jordan VC: Nonisomerizable analogues of (Z)- and (E)-4-hydroxytamoxifen. Synthesis and endocrinological properties of substituted diphenylbenzocycloheptenes. J Med Chem 1988 (31):1285-1290

13   Murphy CS and Jordan VC: Structural components necessary for the antiestrogenic activity of tamoxifen. J Steroid Biochem 1989 (34):407-411

14   Kawamura I, Mizota T, Mukumoto S et al: Antiestrogenic and antitumor effects of droloxifene in experimental breast carcinoma. Arzneim-Forsch 1989 (39):889-893.

15   Toko T, Sugimoto Y, Matsuo KI et al: TAT59. A new triphenylethylene derivative with antitumour activity against hormone dependent tumours. Eur J Cancer 1990 (26):397-404

16   Rowlands MG, Parr IB, McCague R, et al: Variation of the inhibition of calmodulin dependent cyclic AMP phosphodiesterase amongst analogues of tamoxifen; correlations with cytotoxicity. Biochem Pharmacol 1990 (40):283-289

17   Di Salle E, Zaecheo T and Ornati G: Antiestrogenic and antitumour properties of the new triphenylethylene derivative toremifene in the rat. J Steroid Biochem 1990 (36):203-206.

18   Wakeling AE, Dukes M and Bowler J: A potent specific pure antiestrogen with clinical potential. Cancer Res 1991 (51):3867-3873

19   Koike S, Sakai M and Muramatsu M: Molecular cloning and characterisation of rat estrogen receptor cDNA. Nucleic Acids Res 1987 (15):2499-2513

20   Harlow KW, Smith DN, Katzenellenbogen JA et al: Identification of cysteine 530 as the covalent attachment site of an affinity-labelling estrogen (ketononestrol aziridine) and antiestrogen (tamoxifen aziridine) in the human estrogen receptor. J Biol Chem 1989 (264):17476-17485

21   Knabbe C, Lippman ME, Wakefield LM et al: Evidence that transforming growth factor-ß is a hormonally regulated negative growth factor in human breast cancer cells. Cell 1987 (48):417-428

22   Robinson SP and Jordan VC: The paracrine stimulation of MCF-7 cells by MDA-MB-231 cells: possible role in paracrine effects. Eur J Clin Oncol 1989 (25):493-497

23   Osborne CK, Coronado EB and Robinson JP: Human breast cancer in the athymic nude mouse: cytostatic effects of long-term antiestrogen therapy. Eur J Cancer Clin Oncol 1987 (23):1189-1196

24   Lønning PE and Kvinnsland S: Mechanism of action of aminoglutethimide as endocrine therapy of breast cancer. Drugs 1988 (35):685-710

25   Santen RJ, Santner S, Davis B et al: Aminoglutethimide inhibits extraglandular estrogen production in postmenopausal women with breast carcinoma. J Clin Endocrinol Metab 1978 (47):1257-1265

26   Buzdar AU, Powell KC, Legha MD and Blumenschein GR: Treatment of advanced breast cancer with aminoglutethimide after therapy with tamoxifen. Cancer 1982 (50):1708-1712

27   Ali H, Khalaf L, Nicholls PJ, Poole A: Comparison of in vitro and in vivo hemotoxic effects of aminoglutethimide and glutethimide. Toxicol in Vitro 1990 (4):381-383

28 Lien EA, Anker G, Lønning PE et al: Decreased serum concentrations of tamoxifen and its metabolites induced by aminoglutethimide. Cancer Res 1990 (50):5851-5857

29 Van Wauwe JP and Janssen PAJ: Is there a case for P-450 inhibitors in cancer treatment? J Med Chem 1989 (32):2231-2239

30 Haynes BP, Jarman M, Dowsett M et al: Pharmacokinetics and pharmacodynamics of the aromatase inhibitor 3-ethyl-3-(4-pyridyl)piperidine-2,6-dione in patients with postmenopausal breast cancer. Cancer Chemother Pharmacol 1991 (27):367-372

31 Kitawaki J, Yamamoto T, Urabe M et al: Selective aromatase inhibition by pyridoglutethimide, an analogue of aminoglutethimide. Acta Endocrinologica 1990 (122):592-598

32 Dowsett M, Stein RC, Mehta A and Coombes RC: Potency and selectivity of a non-steroidal aromatase inhibitor CGS 16949A in postmenopausal breast cancer patients. Clin Endocrinol 1990 (32):623-624

33 Bhatnagar AS, Haensler A, Schieweck K et al: Highly selective inhibition of estrogen biosynthesis by CGS 20267, a new non-steroidal aromatase inhibitor. J Steroid Biochem Mol Biol 1990 (37):1021-1027

34 Kellis JT, Jr and Vickery LE: The active site of aromatase cytochrome P-450. J Biol Chem 1987 (262):8840-8844

35 Laughton CA, McKenna R, Neidle S et al: Crystallographic and molecular modelling studies on 3-ethyl-3-(4-pyridyl)piperidine-2,6-dione and its butyl analogue, inhibitors of mammalian aromatase. Comparison with natural substrates: prediction of enantioselectivity for N-alkyl derivatives. J Med Chem 1990 (33):2673-2679

36 Banting L, Smith JH, James M et al: structure-activity relationships for non-steroidal inhibitors of aromatase. J Enzyme Inhibition 1988 (2):215-229

37 Brodie AMH, Schwarzel WC, Shaikh AA and Brodie HJ: The effect of an aromatase inhibitor, 4-hydroxy-4-androstene-3,17-dione, on estrogen-dependent processes in reproduction and breast cancer. Endocrinology 1977 (100):1684-1695

38 Dowsett M, Goss PE, Powles TJ et al: Use of the aromatase inhibitor 4-hydroxyandrostenedione in postmenopausal breast cancer: optimization of therapeutic dose and route. Cancer Res 1987 (47):1957-1961

39 Marcotte PA and Robinson CH: Synthesis and evaluation of 10ß-substituted 4-estrene-3,17-diones as inhibitors of human placental microsomal aromatase. Steroids 1982 (39):325-344

40 Lønning PE, Jacobs S, Jones A et al: The influence of CGS 16949A on peripheral aromatisation in breast cancer patients. Br J Cancer 1991 (63):789-793

41 Lipton A, Harvey HA, Derners LM et al: A phase I trial of CGS 16949A, a new aromatase inhibitor. Cancer 1990 (65):1279-1285

42 Santner SJ, Feil PD and Santen RJ: In situ estrogen production via the estrone sulfatase pathway in breast tumours: relative importance versus the aromatase pathway. J Clin Endocrinol Metab 1984 (59):29-133

43 Tolis G, Ackman D, Stellos A et al: Tumor growth inhibition in patients with prostatic carcinoma treated with luteinizing hormone-releasing hormone agonists. Proc Natl Acad Sci USA 1982 (79):1658-1662

44 Dutta AS and Furr BJA: Luteinizing Hormone Releasing Hormone (LHRH) Analogues. Chapter 21. In: Annual Reports in Medicinal Chemistry 20. Academic Press Inc, San Diego 1985, pp203-214

45 Borgmann V, Hardt W, Schmidt-Gollwitzer M et al: Sustained suppression of testosterone production by the luteinizing-hormone-releasing-hormone agonist buserelin in patients with advanced prostatic carcinoma. The Lancet 1982 (i): 1097-1099

46 Smith JA, Jr: New methods of endocrine management of prostatic cancer. J Urol 1987 (137):1-10

47 Habenicht U-F, Schneider MR and El Etreby MF: Effect of the new potent LHRH antagonist antide. J Steroid Biochem Molec Biol 1990 (37):937-942

48 Forti G, Salerno R, Moneti G et al: Three month treatment with a long acting gonadotrophin-releasing hormone agonist of patients with benign prostatic hyperplasia. Effects on tissue androgen concentration, 5α-reductase activity and androgen receptor content. J Clin Endocrinol Metab 1989 (68):461-468

49 Crawford ED: Hormonal Therapy of Prostatic Carcinoma. Defining the Challenge. Cancer 1990 (66):1035-1038

50 Labrie F, Dupont A, Giguere M et al: Benefits of combination therapy with flutamide in patients relapsing after castration. Br J Urol 1988 (61):341-346

51 Labrie F, Dupont A, Cuson L et al: Combination therapy with flutamide and medicinal (LHRH agonist) or surgical castration in advanced prostatic cancer: 7-year clinical experience. J Steroid Biochem Mol Biol 1990 (37):943-960

52 Crawford ED, Blumenstein BA and Goodman PJ: Leuprolide with and without flutamide in advanced prostatic cancer. Cancer 1990 (66):1039-1044

53 Keuppens F, Denis L, Smith P et al: Zoladex and flutamide versus bilateral orchiectomy. A randomized phase III EORTC 30853 study. Cancer 1990 (66):1045-1057

54 Iverson P, Christensen MG, Friis E et al: A phase III trial of Zoladex and flutamide versus orchiectomy in the treatment of patients with advanced carcinoma of the prostate. Cancer 1990 (66):1058-1066

55 Knuth UA, Hano R and Nieschlag E: Effect of flutamide or cyproterone acetate on pituitary and testicular hormones in normal men. J Clin Endocrinol Metab 1984 (59):963-969

56 Neumann F and Töpert M: Pharmacology of antiandrogens. J Urol 1978 (120):180-183

57 Hellman L, Bradlow HL, Freed S et al: The effect of flutamide on testosterone metabolism and the plasma levels of androgens and gonadotrophins. J Clin Endocr Metab 1977 (45):1224-1229

58 Katchen B and Buxbaum S: Disposition of a new, non-steroidal, antiandrogen, α,α,α-trifluoro-2-methyl-4'-nitro-m-propionotoluidide (flutamide) in men following a single oral 200 mg dose. J Clin Endocrinol Metab 1975 (41):373-379

59 Liao S, Howell DK and Chang T-M: Action of a non-steroidal antiandrogen flutamide on the receptor binding and nuclear retention of 5alpha-dihydrostestosterone in rat ventral prostate. Endocrinology 1974 (94):1205-1209

60 Tucker H, Crook JW and Chesterson GJ: Non-steroidal antiandrogens. Synthesis and structure-activity relationships of 3-substituted derivatives of 2-hydroxypropionanilides. J Med Chem 1988 (31):954-959

61 Moguilewsky M, Fiet J, Tournemine C and Raynaud J-P: Pharmacology of an antiandrogen anandron, used as an adjuvant therapy in the treatment of prostatic cancer. J Steroid Biochem 1986 (24):139-146

62 Furr BJA, Valcaccia B, Curry B et al: ICI 176,334: a novel non-steroidal, peripherally selective antiandrogen. J Endocrinol 1987 (113):R7-R9

63 Snyder BW, Winneker RC and Batzold FH: Endocrine profile of Win 49596 in the rat: a novel androgen receptor antagonist. J Steroid Biochem 1989 (33):1127-1132

64 Mahajan DK and Samuels LT: Inhibition of 17,20(17-hydroxyprogesterone)-lyase by progesterone. Steroids 1975 (25):217-227

65 Santen RJ, van den Bossche H, Symoens J et al: Site of action of low dose ketoconazole in androgen biosynthesis in men. J Clin Endocrinol Metab 1983 (57):732-736

66 Dowsett M, Shearer RJ, Ponder BAJ et al: The effect of aminoglutethimide and hydrocortisone, alone and combined, on androgen levels in post-orchiectomy prostatic cancer patients. Br J Cancer 1988 (57):190-192

67 English HJ, Santner SJ, Levine HB and Santen RJ: Inhibitor of testosterone production with ketoconazole alone and in combination with a gonadotrophin releasing hormone analogue in the rat. Cancer Res 1986 (46):38-42

68 Rajfer J, Sikka SC, Riviera F and Handelsman DJ: Mechanism of inhibition of human testicular steroidogenesis by oral ketoconazole. J Clin Endocrinol Metab 1986 (63):1193-1198

69 Bruynseels J, De Coster R, Van Rooy P et al: R75251, a new inhibitor of steroid biosynthesis. The Prostate 1990 (16):345-357

70 Trachtenberg J and Toledo A: Evidence for action in hormone refractory disease. R75251, a novel non-toxic treatment of hormone refractory prostatic cancer. J Urol 1991 (145):Abstr 420

71 McCague R, Rowlands MG, Barrie SE and Houghton J: Inhibition of enzymes of estrogen and androgen biosynthesis by esters of 4-pyridylacetic acid. J Med Chem 1990 (33):3050-3055

72 Laughton CA and Neidle S: Inhibitors of the P450 enzymes aromatase and lyase. Crystallographic and molecular modelling studies suggest structural features of pyridylacetic acid derivatives responsible for differences in enzyme inhibitory activity. J Med Chem 1990 (33): 3055-3060

73 Chung B-C, Picado-Leonard J, Haniu M et al: Cytochrome P450c17 (steroid 17α-hydroxylase/$_{17,20}$ lyase): cloning of human adrenal and testis cDNAs indicates the same gene is expressed in both tissues. Proc Natl Acad Sci USA 1987 (84):407-411

74 Poulos TL, Finzel BC, Gunsalus IC et al: The 2.6-Å crystal structure of Pseudomonas putida cytochrome P-450. J Biol Chem 1985 (260):16122-16130

75 Laughton CA, Neidle S, Zvelebil MJJM and Sternberg MJE: A molecular model for the enzyme cytochrome $P450_{17\alpha}$, a major target for the chemotherapy of prostatic cancer. Biochem Biophys Res Commun 1990 (171):1160-1167

76 Angelastro MR, Laughlin ME, Schatzman GL et al: 17ß-(Cyclopropylamino)androst-5-en-3ß-ol, a selective mechanism based inhibitor of cytochrome $P450_{17\alpha}$ (steroid 17α-hydroxylase/C_{17-20}lyase). Biochem Biophys Res Commun 1989 (162):1571-1577

77 Miller SL, Wright JN, Corina DL and Akhtar M: Mechanistic studies on pregnene side-chain cleavage enzyme (17α-hydroxylase-17,20-lyase) using ^{18}O. J Chem Soc, Chem Commun 1991:157-159

78 Baulieu EE, Lasnitzki I and Robel P: Metabolism of testosterone and action of metabolites on prostate glands grown in organ culture. Nature 1968 (219):1155-1156

79 Petrow V, Wang Y-S and Lack L: Prostatic cancer 1. 6-methylene-4-pregnen-3-ones as irreversible inhibitors of rat prostate Δ^4-3-ketosteroid 5α-reductase. Steroids 1981 (38):121-140

80 Petrow V, Padilla GM, McPhail AT et al: Prostate III - A structural feature characteristic of the rat prostate 5α-reductase active site. J Steroid Biochem 1989 (32):399-407

81 Rasmusson GH, Reynolds GF, Steinberg NG et al: Azasteroids. SAR for inhibition of 5α-reductase and of androgen receptor binding. J Med Chem 1986 (29):2298-2315

82 Kadohama N, Wakisaka M, Kim U et al: Retardation of prostate tumour progression in the Noble rat by 4-methyl-4-aza-steroidal inhibitors of 5alpha-reductase. JNCI 1985 (74):475-486

83 Fair WR, Presti JC Jr, Sogani P et al: Multicenter, randomized, double blind, placebo controlled study to investigate the effect of finasteride (MK-906) on stage D prostate cancer. J Urol 1991 (145) Abstr 419

84 Gormley GJ, Soner E, Rittmaster RS et al: Effects of finasteride (MK-906) a 5α-reductase inhibitor on circulating androgens in male volunteers. J Clin Endocrinol Metab 1990 (70):1136-1141

85 Metcalf BN: Inhibition of steroid 5alpha-reductase. In: Palfreyman MG, McCann PP, Lovenberg W et al (eds) Enzymes as Targets for Drug Design. Academic Press Inc, San Diego 1990, pp 85-100

86 Houston B, Chisholm GD and Habib FK: A kinetic analysis of the 5α-reductases from human prostate and liver. Steroids 1987 (49):355-369

87 Levy MA, Brandt M, Holt DA and Metcalf VW: Interaction between rat prostatic steroid 5alpha-reductase and 3-carboxy-17β-substituted steroids: novel mechanism of enzyme inhibition. J Steroid Biochem 1989 (34):571-575

88 Anderson S and Russell DW: Structure and biochemical properties of cloned and expressed human and rat steroid 5alpha-reductases. Proc Natl Acad Sci USA 1990 (87):3640-3644

89 Liang T, Cascieri MA, Cheung AH et al: Species differences in prostatic steroid 5α-reductases of rat, dog and human. Endocrinology 1985 (117):571-57

90 McCague R: Inhibitors of steroid hormone biosynthesis and action. In: Wilman DEV (ed) Chemistry of Antitumour Agents. Blackie & Son Ltd, Glasgow 1990 pp 234-260

Design of Novel Bioreductive Drugs

Paul Workman

Cancer Research Campaign Beatson Laboratories, CRC Department of Medical Oncology, University of Glasgow, Alexander Stone Building, Garscube Estate, Switchback Road, Bearsden, Glasgow G61 1BD, United Kingdom

There is currently a great need and indeed considerable enthusiasm to search for new drug molecules with improved therapeutic selectivity in the major solid tumours. One approach is to screen novel structures for activity in biologically relevant models. This is the new approach taken by the United States National Cancer Institute which places much emphasis on panels of human cell lines to test natural products *in vitro*. An alternative strategy is to identify differences in biochemical structure and function between normal and neoplastic cells and to develop agents to exploit these novel targets on a rational basis. There are many new and exciting possibilities. The elaboration of agents which interfere with oncogene function, growth factors and their receptors, transmembrane signal transduction and so on, are good examples. Considerable attention is also being directed towards another exploitable target based on the aberrant physiology of solid tumours: cellular hypoxia [1].

The Biology of Hypoxia

Hypoxic cells are those existing at an oxygen concentration which is suboptimal for cell growth and metabolism, but nevertheless sufficient to maintain viability. Thus, these cells are at an intermediate oxygen tension between the well-oxygenated cells known as the oxic population and those cells at very low oxygen tensions known as the anoxic necrotic population.

There are actually 2 types of hypoxia in solid tumours (Fig. 1). The classic model is known as chronic or diffusion-limited hypoxia [2,3]. The diffusion distance of molecular oxygen through tissue is limited by metabolic consumption to 150-200 microns (around one-fifth of a millimetre). Cells at about this distance from the nearest capillary will become hypoxic, and this may persist over a period of hours to days. Cells which are even further from capillaries become so anoxic that they die, forming areas of necrosis. Chronically hypoxic cells are not only deficient in oxygen, they may also be starved of glucose and other nutrients, as well as developing a surplus of metabolic waste products.

There is also a second and more acute type of hypoxia [4,5]. This results from the intermittent opening and closing of tumour blood vessels, producing a local and more transient shortage of oxygen, with a time scale of seconds to minutes. This type of hypoxia is also known as perfusion-limited hypoxia.

It will be clear from this brief description that the biology of tumour hypoxia is very closely linked to the biology to tumour vasculature. The existence of chronic and acute hypoxia in solid tumours results from the fact that the distribution, structure and function of their vasculature are different from normal tissues. Tumour cell growth frequently outstrips the development of adequate supportive vessels, and these in turn may be grossly abnormal in appearance and performance.

Hypoxia and Resistance

Cells treated with X-rays in the absence of oxygen are uniformly 2-3 times more resistant

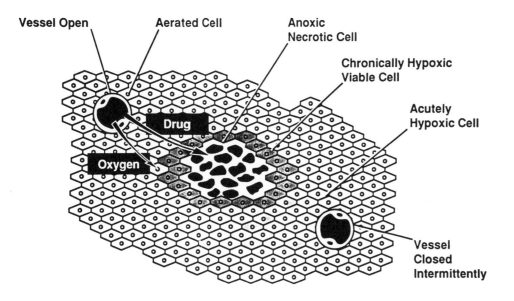

Fig. 1. Two types of hypoxia in solid tumours. *Chronic hypoxia*, as in the classic Tomlinson-Gray model, is caused by the disorganised and rapid growth of the tumour exhausting the supportive vasculature. The diffusion of oxygen through tissue is restricted by its consumption by respiring cells. Cells close to functioning capillaries are well oxygenated, or *normoxic*, and therefore fully viable. With increasing distance from the vessel, the oxygen concentration falls. Beyond about 200 µM, the oxygen level is insufficient to support viability and the *anoxic* cells become necrotic. Cells which exist at the interface between normoxic and anoxic cells are known as *hypoxic*. These have an oxygen level which is low but nevertheless sufficient to allow cells to remain viable. *Acute hypoxia* develops as a consequence of the sequential opening and closing of tumour vessels. When a vessel closes the surrounding cells will rapidly consume the available oxygen and become hypoxic. On reopening, the same cells will regain normoxic status. Acute hypoxia is more transient than chronic hypoxia.

to cell killing than fully oxic ones [3]. Known in radiobiology as the Oxygen Effect, this arises because molecular oxygen is able to interact with short-lived radicals in DNA, leading to irreversible fixation of the damage. This happens in a way which is competitive with radioprotective thiols, such as glutathione, which act to restore the damage.

To give an idea of the concentrations involved, a concentration of 0.25% (1.5 mm Hg) oxygen moves the radiation survival curve halfway towards the fully aerated sensitivity, while at 2% (12 mm Hg) oxygen the shift in response is essentially complete. Hypoxia defined in this way is known as Radiobiological Hypoxia. There is considerable evidence to implicate Radiobiological Hypoxia in radiotherapy treatment failure in such sites as cervix, head and neck and bladder cancer [1]. Venous blood has an oxygen tension of 20-40 mm Hg and most normal tissues will be in this range.

In addition to affecting the response to radiation, Radiobiological Hypoxia can also bring about resistance to various conventional anticancer agents, for example bleomycin and some alkylating agents like melphalan. This may arise through impaired vascular delivery to hypoxic cells, from induction of a non-cycling cell kinetic status, or the involvement of molecular oxygen in the mechanism of action of the drug. Hypoxia can also lead to the expression of "oxygen-regulated proteins" which may affect drug response, and to dihydrofolate reductase gene amplification, causing methotrexate resistance [6]. Changes in the expression of growth factor receptors are also seen.

It will be clear from this discussion that tumour hypoxia can be perceived as an obstacle to cancer therapy.

Strategies to Circumvent Tumour Hypoxia

Probably the most successful technique to overcome tumour hypoxia in clinical radiotherapy is fractionated treatment. This works through re-oxygenation of the tumour between treatments. Nevertheless, there is good evidence that hypoxic cells remain limiting.

Experimental techniques to improve oxygen delivery to tumours include the use of hyperbaric oxygen chambers, perfluorochemical carriers and transfusion, together with haemoglobin and blood flow modifying agents [1].

However, the greatest interest has been in the development of chemicals which can take the place of oxygen in radiosensitising hypoxic cells - these are the so-called oxygen-mimetic or electron-affinic radiosensitisers. Such agents have the advantage of ease of use and ready diffusion into hypoxic regions.

Nitroimidazole Radiosensitisers

Whereas a range of electron affinic chemical structures are effective sensitisers of hypoxic cells *in vitro*, animal work has shown that nitroimidazoles are ideal radiosensitisers *in vivo*, particularly in terms of metabolic stability, delivery to hypoxic cells and host toxicity. For reviews of this extensive field see references 1 and 7.

The 5-nitroimidazole radiosensitiser metronidazole entered clinical trial. However, these agents have rather weak potency compared to the 2-nitroimidazoles such as misonidazole (see Fig. 2 for structure). Although there has been some evidence of clinical radiosensitisation by misonidazole, progress with this agent was marred by dose-limiting neurotoxi-

city. This led to the development of the 2 analogues currently in clinical trial, namely etanidazole (SR 2508) and pimonidazole (Ro 03-8799) (Fig. 2). Etanidazole has the major advantage of exclusion from nervous tissues [8], and doses 3 times those of misonidazole can be given to patients for the same degree of peripheral neuropathy and without central neurotoxicity [9]. Pimonidazole is a more potent agent, and accumulates in tissue by virtue of the basic piperidine function [10,11]. Randomised phase III trials in head and neck (etanidazole) and cervix cancer (pimonidazole) have been carried out, but the results appear to be disappointing. It may be that the achievable drug concentrations were insufficient for activity in the case of etanidazole. The deleterious effects of pimonidazole may be due to the decrease in blood flow noted in mouse tumours. Perhaps surprisingly, a low electron affinity 5-nitroimidazole, nimorazole, does appear to be active in clinical studies.

At the laboratory level, the most promising approach has been the development of very potent "mixed-function" sensitisers containing both the sensitising nitro-group and an alkylating (e.g. aziridine) function. The lead compound RSU 1069 [12] disappointingly showed dose-limiting gastrointestinal toxicity [13]; however, the derivative RB 6145 [14] contains a masked aziridine moiety, is less toxic and is now in preclinical development (Fig. 2, see later).

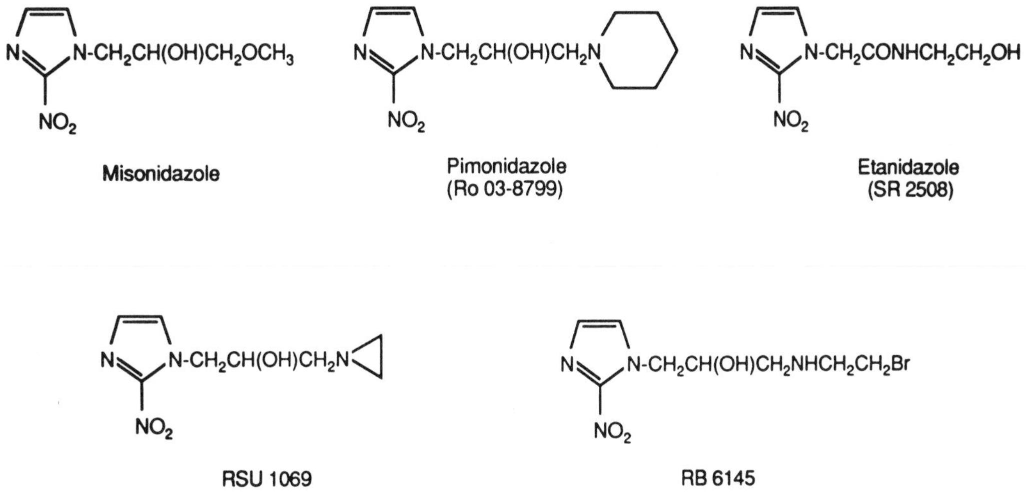

Fig. 2. Structures of 2-nitroimidazole radiosensitisers and bioreductive hypoxic cell cytotoxins

Mechanisms of Radiosensitisation and Chemosensitisation

The principal mechanism of radiosensitisation involves the fast free radical mechanism mentioned earlier. However, additional mechanisms are now known to operate, notably including the "preincubation effect" which requires prolonged exposure before radiation [15]. This necessitates cellular metabolism of the sensitiser, leading to effects such as glutathione depletion and inhibition of DNA repair. These 2 factors also bring about sensitisation of hypoxic cells to some conventional chemotherapeutic agents, most notably alkylating agents like melphalan and some nitrosoureas [16].

Bioreductive Cytotoxins and Bioreductive Metabolism

During the development of nitroimidazoles it was recognised that these agents express the ability to kill radiobiologically hypoxic cells much more efficiently than oxic ones [16]. This is in fact a common feature of chemicals able to undergo Bioreductive Metabolism to generate toxic drug metabolites [17]. The preferential toxicity towards hypoxic cells is a result of the absence of oxygen which can usually reverse this activation pathway. On the other hand, this reversal usually generates active oxygen radicals like superoxide - such radicals can also result in toxicity to aerobic cells, but in most cases this is less than that due to active drug metabolites, because of the activity of protective enzymes such as superoxide dismutase and catalase which detoxify oxygen radicals. A number of nitro group-containing antimicrobial agents, for example metronidazole, benznidazole, nitrofurazone and nitrofurantoin, also exert their selectivity through a similar mechanism - formation of toxic drug metabolites.

Main Classes of Bioreductive Anticancer Drugs

The main types of bioreductive anticancer drugs [7] have traditionally been the nitro compounds mentioned earlier (Fig. 2) and the quinone agents of which the prototype is the naturally occurring antibiotic mitomycin C [18] and another example is EO9 [19] (Fig. 3). Until just recently, little progress was made in the identification of new bioreductive drug classes. A significant breakthrough was achieved, however, with the discovery of the benzotriazine di-N-oxides as potent and

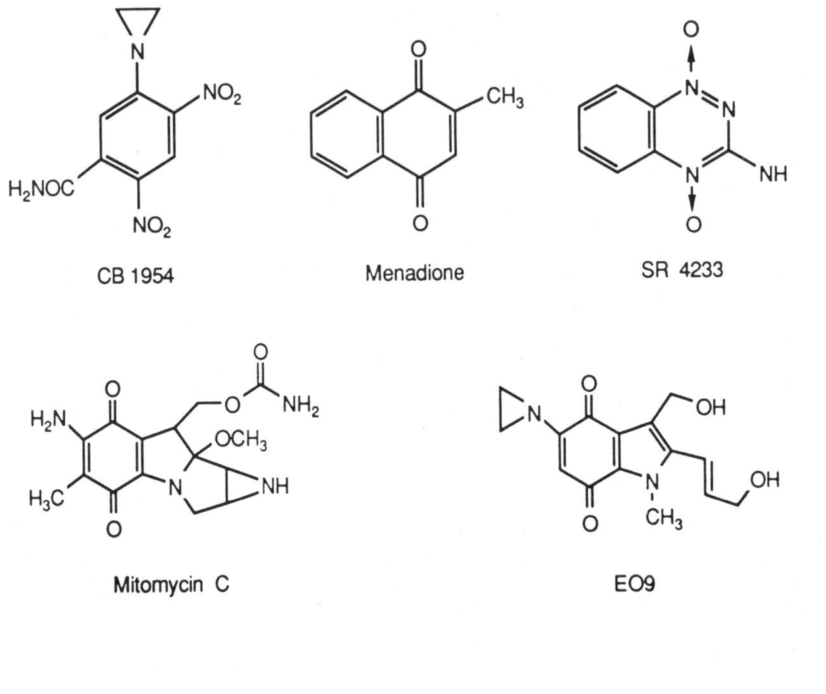

CB 1954

Menadione

SR 4233

Mitomycin C

EO9

Fig. 3. Structures of various bioreductive hypoxic cell cytotoxins

specific hypoxic cell cytotoxins [20]. These are exemplified by the lead compound WIN 59075 (SR 4233) (Fig. 3). Theoretical models support the intuitive view that it is likely to be more effective to kill the hypoxic cell population of a tumour than to sensitise it to radiation [21].

The active metabolites which are formed from bioreductive drugs under hypoxic conditions have been described in some detail [17]. With nitro compounds these include the nitroradical anion (1 electron reduced), nitroso (2 electron) and hydroxylamine (4 electron). In the case of the quinone alkylating agents like mitomycin C and EO9, 1 electron reduction forms the semiquinone free radical and 2 electron reduction produces the hydroquinone. Both processes activate the 2 or more latent alkylating functions of the prodrug molecule resulting in the crosslinking of the Watson-Crick DNA double helix. This also occurs with the "dual-function" nitroimidazoles but in most cases a DNA-monoadduct is formed from nitro compounds. N-oxide drugs are different in that 1 electron reduction forms an oxidising nitroxide radical which abstracts hydrogen from bases in DNA, creating both single and double strandbreaks without forming drug-DNA adducts.

In Vitro Cytotoxicity Screening for Bioreductive Agents

In terms of selecting a bioreductive drug to take forward to clinical development, the traditional approach has been to pursue the goal of maximising the differential cytotoxicity between hypoxic and oxic cells. This type of testing has usually been carried out using EMT6 mouse mammary tumour cells, V79 fibroblasts or Chinese hamster ovary cells with either clonogenic assay or tetrazolium dye reduction as endpoints [22]. Typical results are illustrated in Figure 4. Some well established hypoxic/oxic differentials are around 10 for misonidazole, 1-3 for mitomycin C and 50-100 for both WIN 59075 and RSU 1069/RB 6145 (for structures see Figs. 2 and 3). Thus, WIN 59075 and RSU 1069/RB 6145 emerge as especially "clean" (i.e., high specificity) hypoxic cell cytotoxins. In addition, re-

cent studies have shown the indoloquinone EO9, related in structure to mitomycin C, to exhibit not only improved potency, but also a much higher hypoxic/oxic differential than is normally seen with quinones. This is, however, less than can be obtained for WIN 59075 and RSU 1069.

It is appropriate to add a couple of important caveats at this point. These concern the more variable nature of hypoxic cell cytotoxicity as against hypoxic cell radiosensitisation. Almost certainly because of the requirement for cell metabolism in hypoxic cell cytotoxicity, the differentials obtained do not appear to be as consistent across cell lines. For example, with WIN 59075 rather lower hypoxic/oxic cytotoxicity differentials are seen in certain human cell strains. This makes it more difficult to envisage an equal effect of hypoxic cell cytotoxins across various tumour types. Moreover, such observations emphasise the potential pitfall of relying on a single cell type for drug screening. The reason for this biological diversity of response probably lies in the heterogeneity of expression of bioreductive enzymes (see later). The activities of enzymes protecting aerobic cells from oxidative stress are probably also important, together with the levels of DNA repair enzymes.

The second cautionary point to introduce here is that the concentrations of oxygen considered as "oxic" and "hypoxic" by radiobiologists and radiation oncologists may not be exactly the same as those modulating response to different hypoxic cell cytotoxins. In particular, there may be a more stringent requirement for lack of oxygen to bring about optimal metabolism and hypoxic cell killing.

Strategies for in Vitro Evaluation

There is no unified consensus as to the appropriate in vivo evaluation strategy for bioreductives which appear promising in the in vitro assays derived above. This remains a subject for debate. A combination of various model systems is likely to be of greater value than any single one.

In vivo testing should include evaluation against clinically relevant tumour models. Hypoxia-inducing drugs can be used to po-

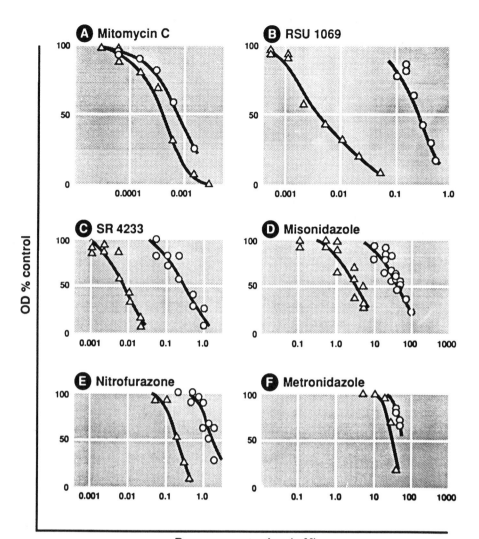

Fig. 4. Differential cytotoxicity of various bioreductive agents in hypoxic (triangles) versus oxic (circles) cells. The results are redrawn from reference 22. Note that the dual-function 2-nitroimidazole RSU 1069 and the benzotriazine-di-*N*-oxide SR 4233 (WIN 59075) show especially large differentials in these V79 Chinese hamster fibroblasts.

tentiate the activity of hypoxic cell cytotoxins by increasing the depth or extent of hypoxia. These include blood flow modifiers, such as hydralazine and flavone acetic acid, and oxyhaemoglobin dissociation modifiers like BW12C. The results seem to be quite variable with these agents, and it can be argued that although interesting mechanistically, modifying agents may not be ideal in screening for bioreductives *in vivo*. Pharmacokinetic properties, particularly tumour penetration, should be considered an important factor. The potential complexity of pharmacokinetic behaviour was illustrated in studies with RB 6145 [23] and EO9 [24]. Probably the most crucial features of an *in vivo* model are the degree of hypoxia and the expression of reductive enzymes.

Enzymology of Bioreduction

The importance of understanding the enzymes involved in bioreduction is rapidly gaining widespread recognition [16,25]. It is clear that many different enzymes are involved in the production of toxic bioreduction products. Multiple enzymes can be involved in the metabolism of a given agent. Different enzymes can be predominantly involved in early versus later steps of a multi-step reaction pathway. For some compounds it has been proposed that obligate 2-electron (as against 1-electron) donating enzymes may be protective.

Enzymes known to be involved in bioreductive metabolism include cytochrome P-450, cytochrome P-450 reductase, xanthine oxidase, aldehyde oxidase, carbonyl reductase, and DT-diaphorase, together with mitochondrial reductases and probably many others as well. Examples of the complexity of the picture are provided by our own studies with the 2-nitroimidazole benznidazole and the benzotriazine di-*N*-oxide WIN 59075. Mouse liver microsomes were used as a rich source of bioreductive enzymes. The results showed that for benznidazole cytochrome P450 reductase was predominantly involved in the early stages of the bioactivation pathway (e.g., formation of the nitro radical anion), while cytochrome P450 was preferentially involved in later stages leading to amine formation [26]. In the case of WIN 59075, cytochrome P450 reductase catalyses 30% of microsomal WIN 59075 reduction while cytochrome P450 is responsible for the remaining 70% [27]. Our more recent work has shown that specific isoenzymes of the cytochrome P450 multigene family are preferentially involved - particularly dexamethasone-inducible 2B and 2C forms [28].

With mitomycin C, cytochrome P450 plays only a minor part, apparently stimulating reduction by cytochrome P450 reductase which has a critical role [17]. Recent results suggest that DT-diaphorase, like cytochrome P450, cannot bioactivate mitomycin C except under low pH conditions [29-31]. Although it is possible that low pH micro environments may occur, the current view is that the average intracellular pH is alkaline: thus the significance of DT-diaphorase with respect to mitomycin C remains unclear. DT-diaphorase is, however, a major enzyme in the activation of the interesting bioreductive agent CB 1954 [32] (Fig. 2) as well as the indoloquinone EO9 [30,33].

Enzyme-Directed Bioreductive Drug Development

Until recently the synthesis of bioreductive agents for screening in oxic versus hypoxic cells was dominated by considerations of redox potential and to a lesser extent lipophilicity and charge. However, these factors cannot routinely predict for bioreductive cytotoxicity, particularly *in vivo*. The growing appreciation of the key role of bioreductive enzymes has led to the concept of enzyme-directed bioreductive drug development [25]. We have proposed that the antitumour selectivity of bioreductive agents could be enhanced not only by tumour hypoxia, but in addition by increased expression of key reductase enzymes in cancer cells. We have further suggested that even greater selectivity might be gained by tailor-making drugs to be activated specifically by particular reductases that are expressed at high levels in tumours.

Progress towards this goal has been made with DT-diaphorase. Particular alterations in the chemical structure of mitomycin C, EO9, diaziquone and CB 1954 produce startling differences in the ability of these agents to undergo reductive metabolism by the enzyme [31,34]. For example, in the case of EO9 changes to the aziridine group have a marked effect. Moreover, the rate of metabolism correlates with cytotoxicity in the EO9 series.

It is too early to assess the likely success of this approach to developing new and improved bioreductive agents. However, an elucidation of the molecular enzymology [35] of particular bioreductive agents is also likely to have an impact on the choice of human tumour types or even individual patients for bioreductive therapy.

Enzyme Profiling

We currently know relatively little about the comparative expression of bioreductive enzymes in human tumour versus normal tissues. In fact, this is also true for the *in vitro* and *in vivo* tumour models which are used to select bioreductive agents. It seems clear that the development and clinical use of these drugs would be more rational if we had further information available to us.

Clearly, if we knew that a particular drug was activated especially well by certain enzymes, it would be appropriate to evaluate this agent (and its derivatives) in tumours rich in this enzyme. Furthermore, it would also be sensible to target the clinical use of the drug to those tumours which also expressed high levels of enzyme activity. This might be a certain class

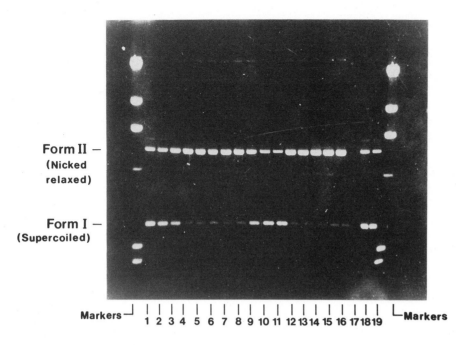

Form II —
(Nicked
relaxed)

Form I —
(Supercoiled)

Markers ⌐ | | | | | | | | | | | | | | | | | | | ⌐ Markers
1 2 3 4 5 6 7 8 9 10 11 12 13 14 15 16 17 18 19

Fig. 5. Effects of increasing concentrations of EO9, dicoumarol and superoxide dismutase on the damage induced in pBR 322 plasmid DNA as a result of reduction of EO9 catalysed by DT-diaphorase purified from rat UK Walker 256 mammary tumour cells. Incubations (60 min) contained 2 mM NADH, 0.14% bovine serum albumin and 1.6 µg plasmid pBR 322 DNA in a final volume of 100 µl of 100 mM sodium phosphate buffer, pH 7.4. Unless stated otherwise, the incubations also contained 12 Units of DT-diaphorase and 100 µM EO9. Reactions were stopped by addition of 20 µl to 5 µl of stop buffer and a 20 µl aliquot was electrophoresed in a horizontal 0.8% (w/v) agarose gel. Lanes 1-6 show the effect of increasing EO9 concentrations (0, 2, 10, 50, 100 and 200 µM). Lanes 7-11 show the effects of increasing dicoumarol concentrations (0, 1, 5, 10 and 100 µM). Lanes 12-16 show the effects of increasing amounts of superoxide dismutase (0, 25, 50, 100 and 200 Units per 100 µl). Lanes 18 and 19 are controls omitting enzyme and NADH, respectively. Lane 17 is blank. Molecular weight markers are included in the 2 lanes at the extreme left and right. This experiment shows that reduction of EO9 by DT-diaphorase causes DNA strand breaks. These are blocked by the DT-diaphorase inhibitor dicoumarol. The lack of inhibition by superoxide dismutase suggests direct alkylation of DNA by activated drug.

of tumours, say colon cancer, or particular individuals.

Let us consider the specific example of DT-diaphorase and the indoloquinone EO9. We have shown not only that EO9 is activated to DNA-damaging species by DT-diaphorase (ref. 33 and Fig. 5), but also that it exhibits preferential antitumour activity against a human colon tumour cell line *in vitro* and a mouse colon tumour *in vivo*, both of which exhibit much higher DT-diaphorase activities compared to their comparatively unresponsive counterparts [36,37]. We might predict, therefore, that human tumours similarly rich in DT-diaphorase would be the most likely to respond to EO9.

As well as being elevated in a number of chemical carcinogenesis models, DT-diaphorase has been reported to show a high level of expression in some, but not all, human colon, breast, lung and liver tumours [31]. Thus, these may be good targets for EO9 therapy.

Although the situation is less well defined than it is for EO9, WIN 59075 may be especially effective in tumours with high levels of cytochrome P450 and cytochrome P450 re-

ductase. Significant levels of cytochrome P450 2C and 3A have been found in human breast and colorectal tumours. Conversely, there is evidence that WIN 59075 may be detoxified by DT-diaphorase because the 4 and 6 electron reduction pathway seems to bypass the active 1 electron reduced nitroxide radical [38]. So it is possible that, other things being equal, high diaphorase tumours may be comparatively resistant to WIN 59075.

It is quite possible that the tumour reductase enzyme profile will change in response to therapy with bioreductive enzymes. In particular, it would be anticipated that we would see a down-regulation of activating enzymes and/or an up-regulation of protective enzymes. As an example, a cell line made resistant to mitomycin C *in vitro* exhibited a 3-fold decrease in the expression of the activating enzyme cytochrome P450 reductase [39].

With further information of this type it seems possible that the bioreductive enzyme profile of human tumours could be used to guide the choice of bioreductive antitumour agent. Ideally this would be done alongside a measurement of tumour hypoxia.

Prevalence of Hypoxia in Tumours

Virtually all experimental animal tumours contain radiobiologically hypoxic cells. The proportion may be as high as 50%, but it is commonly 10-15% [40]. It seems likely that a similar picture will apply in human solid tumours. Until recently, the evidence was largely indirect, including for example histological structure and haemoglobin status [1]. This was supported by some microelectrode work and confirmed further more recently with smaller and more sophisticated microelectrodes. In a study of 15 breast cancer patients the median oxygen partial pressure (pO_2) was 30 mm Hg compared with 65 mm Hg in the normal breast tissue of patients [41]. Moreover, 6 of 15 breast cancer patients contained areas of tissue with pO_2 values of 0-2.5 mm Hg, whereas in the normal breast values of 12.5 mm Hg and below were not seen. Hence 40% of the tumours looked at continued hypoxic areas with pO_2 levels which would give less than half-maximal radiosensitivity. Similar results have also been obtained in cervix tumours and, moreover, patients with the more hypoxic tumours did worse in terms of radiation response than those with the better oxygenated tumours [Vaupel P, personal communication and in press]. Thus, it seems certain that hypoxic cells do occur at a level equal to or greater than that of the 15-30% in many rodent and xenograft tumours - experimental models in which the therapeutic advantages of bioreductive drugs have been clearly demonstrated.

Techniques are now under development which should allow hypoxic cells to be identified non-invasively. Particular promise is being shown by fluorinated derivatives of nitroimidazoles, the retention of which in hypoxic tumour cells can be visualised by magnetic resonance spectroscopy (MRS, with natural abundance 19F) [42,43] or positron emission tomography (PET, with isotope 18F) [44]. The likelihood of success with these approaches is shown by the excellent results obtained in model systems, together with the demonstrated accumulation of 14C-labelled misonidazole in biopsy specimens from human cancers [45]. The binding of fluorinated nitroimidazoles to hypoxic cells depends on the same biochemical events which activate nitroimidazole bioreductive agents like RSU 1069 and RB 6145 [16]. Because of this we might expect that the application of these molecular probes for hypoxia may be especially suited to use with bioreductive drugs, particularly perhaps nitroimidazole-based agents but hopefully other classes and radiation as well.

Bioreductive Agents in Combination Therapy

It is important to emphasise that bioreductive drugs may not necessarily exert significant activity as single agents. A "clean" bioreductive would be expected to sterilise the hypoxic cells in the tumour, but may not eradicate the oxic cells. An exception will be if the active metabolite is reasonably diffusible. Another is where the bioreductive agents are not quite so specific for hypoxic cells (e.g., mitomycin C and EO9) than is the case with WIN 59075 and RB 6145. However, the general specificity of bioreductive agents for hypoxic cells means that in vivo testing should incorporate studies of the bioreductive in combination with treatments which will kill oxic cells. This might be radiation, conventional cytotoxics like cyclophosphamide, cisplatin and doxorubicin, or perhaps even biologicals and targeted radiotherapy.

Clinical Trials

It follows from the preceding section that clinical testing, perhaps beginning at the phase II level, should involve bioreductives (B) in combination with other therapies. Possible combinations include B + radiotherapy; B + chemotherapy; B + hypoxia inducing agents; and B + hyperthermia.

A variety of tumour sites might be investigated. The most obvious ones from the point of view of hypoxia-limited radiation therapy include head and neck, cervix and brain cancer, and probably also bladder, prostate, lung and melanoma. However, most other tumours including breast and colon cancer will also be of interest and a variety of combinations and protocols could be included. As mentioned earlier, wherever possible measurements of tumour hypoxia and enzyme profile should be carried out. Assays for reduced metabolites in tumour biopsies would also be extremely valuable.

Strengths and Weaknesses of the Bioreductive Approach

A major strength is that this represents a rational attempt to exploit a known Achilles' heel of solid tumours. It seems highly likely to many experimentalists and clinicians that hypoxic cells do limit response to at least some extent in many situations. A good, well-tolerated bioreductive drug should therefore have an excellent chance of finding a role to play in combination chemotherapy or combined modality treatment of various tumours. Because bioreductive drugs are designed to exploit a know "defect" in tumours, there is an excellent opportunity to carry out mechanistic studies as part of the clinical development. As a result, the power of the clinical trials as hypothesis-testing experiments will be enormously increased.

A weakness in a sense is that demonstration of efficacy may well require randomised phase II or even phase III studies. However, most new anticancer agents in development will eventually be used in combinations, and this should not be seen as a serious obstacle. On the other hand, the potential for interacting or additive toxicities should be appreciated at an early stage.

It is probably not a weakness that several bioreductive drugs are currently being developed at the same time. This is because investigator interest is high and because the different agents may prove to be appropriate for different uses, for example according to the degree of hypoxia and/or the bioreductive enzyme spectrum in a given tumour. Sequential use of different bioreductive agents has been proposed in response to a drug-induced alteration in enzyme profile [16].

Concluding Remarks

A number of interesting bioreductive agents are now in development. Both the benzotriazine di-N-oxide WIN 59075 and the indoloquinone EO9 have recently entered clinical trials. RB 6145, or more probably an enantiomer thereof, is likely to go forward. At least 2 mitomycin C analogues (BMY 25067 and KW 2149) are in phase I. Other new agents such as GBJ 584 [46], fused pyrazine mono-N-oxides like RB 90003X (Stratford IJ, personal communication) and N-oxide bioreductive prodrug derivatives of DNA-affinic anthraquinones typified by AQ4N [47], will also be monitored with considerable interest. Other new bioreductive agents are being developed by various groups and it seems likely that the rational design element will continue to gain prominence. We are not yet in a position to create a designer bioreductive prodrug from scratch, and an enlightened medicinal chemistry approach coupled to sensible test systems and a molecular enzymology dimension appears to have the greatest potential at the present time. However, X-ray crystal structures for bioreductive enzymes, if forthcoming, in tandem with advanced computational chemistry techniques would add an extra dimension to the current strategies.

The bioreductive drug approach is based on a firm scientific rationale. A lot of thought is going into refining their development. Clinical studies must be designed with mechanism of action closely in mind, so that these interesting drugs can be used optimally and in order that the maximum amount of information can be obtained.

Acknowledgement

Thanks to Margaret Jenkins for skilful preparation of the manuscript.

REFERENCES

1   Coleman CN: Hypoxia in tumors: A paradigm for the approach to biochemical and physiologic heterogeneity. JNCI 1988 (80):310-317

2   Thomlinson RH and Gray LH: The histological structure of some human lung cancers and the possible implications for radiotherapy. Br J Cancer 1955 (9): 539-549

3   Hall EH: Radiobiology for the Radiologist. Harper and Row, New York 1988

4   Brown JM: Evidence for acutely hypoxic cells in mouse tumours, and a possible mechanism for reoxygenation. Br J Radiol 1979 (52):650-656

5   Horseman MR and Overgaard J: Overcoming tumour radiation resistance resulting from acute hypoxia. Eur J Cancer 1992 (28A):717-718

6   Rice GC, Hoy CA and Schimke RT: Transient hypoxia enhances the frequency of dihydrofolate gene amplification in Chinese hamster ovary cells. Proc Natl Acad Sci 1986 (83):5978-5982

7   Wasserman TH, Sieman D and Workman P (eds): The Seventh International Conference on Chemical Modifiers of Cancer Treatment. Int J Radiat Oncol Biol Phys 1992 (22, Nos. 3 and 4):391-825

8   Brown JM and Workman P Partition coefficient as a guide to the development of radiosensitizers which are less toxic than misonidazole. Radiat Res 1980 (82):171-190

9   Coleman CN, Wasserman TH, Urtasun RC, Halsey J, Hirst VK, Hancock S and Phillips TL: Phase I trial of the hypoxic cell radiosensitizer SR 2508: the results of the five to six week schedule. Int J Radiat Oncol Biol Phys 1986 (12):1105-1108

10 Saunders MI, Anderson PJ, Bennett MH, Dische S, Minchington A, Stratford MRL and Tothill M: The clinical testing of Ro 03-8799 - pharmacokinetics, toxicology, tissue and tumor concentrations. Int J Radiat Oncol Biol Phys 1984 (10):1759-1763

11 Roberts JT, Bleehen NM, Walton MI and Workman P: A clinical phase I toxicity study of Ro 03-8799: plasma, urine, tumour and normal brain pharmacokinetics. Br J Radiol 1986 (59):107-116

12 Stratford IJ, O'Neill P, Sheldon PW, Silver ARJ, Walling JM and Adams GE: RSU 1069, a nitroimidazole containing an aziridine group. Biochem Pharmacol 1986 (35):105-109

13 Horwich A, Holliday SB, Deacon JM, Peckham MJ: A toxicity and pharmacokinetic study in man of the hypoxic cell radiosensitizer RSU 1069. Br J Radiol 1986 (59):1238-1243

14 Jenkins TC, Naylor MA, O'Neill P, Threadgill MD, Cole S, Stratford IJ, Adams GE, Fielden EM, Suto MJ and Stier MA: Synthesis and evaluation 1-[3-(2-haloethylamino)propyl)-2-nitroimidazoles as pro-drugs of RSU 1069 and its analogs, which are radiosensitizers and bioreductively activated cytotoxins. J Med Chem 1990 (33):2603-2610

15 Hall EJ, Astor MA, Biaglow J and Parham JC: The enhanced sensitivity of mammalian cells to killing by X-rays after prolonged exposure to several nitroimidazoles. Int J Radiat Oncol Biol Phys 1982 (8):447-451

16 Stratford IJ, Adams GE, Horsman MR, Kandaiya S, Rajaratnam S, Smith E and Williamson C: The interaction of misonidazole with radiation, chemotherapeutic agents, or heat. Cancer Clin Trials 1980 (3):231-236

17 Workman P: Bioreductive mechanisms. Int J Rad Oncol Biol Phys 1992 (22):631-637

18 Sartorelli AC: Therapeutic attack of solid tumours. Cancer Res 1988 (48):775-778

19 Oostveen EA and Speckamp WN: Mitomycin C analogues 1. Indoloquinones as potential bisalkylating agents. Tetrahedron 1987 (43):255-262

20 Zeman EM, Brown JM, Lemmon MJ, Hirst VK and Lee WW: SR 4233: a new bioreductive agent with high selective toxicity for hypoxic mammalian cells. Int J Radiat Oncol Biol Phys 1986 (12):1239-1242

21 Brown JM and Koong A: Therapeutic advantage of hypoxic cells in tumors: a theoretical study. JNCI 1991 (83):178-185

22 Stratford IJ and Stephens MA: The differential hypoxic cell cytotoxicity of bioreductive agents determined *in vitro* by the MTT assay. Int J Radiat Oncol Biol Phys 1989 (16):973-976

23 Binger M and Workman P: Pharmacokinetic contribution to the improved therapeutic selectivity of a novel bromoethylamino prodrug (RB 6145) of the mixed-function hypoxic cell sensitizer/cytotoxin alpha-(1-aziridinomethyl)-2-nitro-1*H*-imidazole-1-ethanol (RSU 1069). Cancer Chemother Pharmacol 1991 (29):37-47

24 Workman P, Binger M and Kooistra KL: Pharmacokinetics, distribution and metabolism of the novel bioreductive alkylating indoloquinone EO9 in rodents. Int J Radiat Oncol Biol Phys 1992 (22):713-716

25 Workman P and Walton MI: Enzyme-directed bioreductive drug development. In: Adams GE, Breccia A, Fielden EM, Wardman P (eds) Selective Activation of Drugs by Redox Processes. Plenum Press, New York 1991 pp 173-191

26 Walton MI and Workman P: Nitroimidazole bioreductive metabolism: quantitation and characterization of mouse tissue benznidazole nitroreductase *in vivo* and *in vitro*. Biochem Pharmacol 1987 (36):887-896

27 Walton MI and Workman P: Enzymology of the reductive bioactivation of SR 4233: A novel benzotriazine di-*N*-oxide hypoxic cell cytotoxin. Biochem Pharmac 1990 (39):1735-1742

28 Workman P, Walton MI, Wolf CR, Hemingway S and Riley RJ: Cytochrome P450s and cytochrome P450 reductase are the major enzymes in the reduction of the bioreductive SR 4233 (WIN 59075) by mouse liver microsomes. Proc Am Assoc Cancer Res 1992 (33):526

29 Siegel D, Gibson NW, Preusch PC and Ross D: Metabolism of mitomycin C by NAD(P)H: (quinone acceptor) oxidoreductase: role in mitomycin C-induced DNA damage and cytotoxicity in human colon carcinoma cells. Cancer Res 1990 (50):7483-7489

30 Walton MI, Suggett N and Workman P: The role of human and rodent DT-diaphorase in the reductive

metabolism of hypoxic cell cytotoxins. Int J Radiat Oncol Biol Phys 1992 (22):643-647

31 Riley R and Workman P: DT-diaphorase and cancer chemotherapy. Biochem Pharmac 1992 (43):1657-1669

32 Knox RJ, Boland MP, Friedlos F, Coles B, Southan CS, Roberts JJ: The nitroreductase enzyme in Walker cells that activates 5-(aziridin-1-yl)-4-hydroxylamino-2-nitrobenzamide is a form of NAD(P)H dehydrogenase (quinone) (EC 1.6.99.2). Biochem Pharmacol 1988 (37):4671-4677

33 Walton MI, Smith PJ and Workman P: The role of NAD(P)H: quinone reductase (EC 1.6.99.2, DT-diaphorase) in the reductive bioactivation of the novel indoloquinone antitumour agent EO9. Cancer Communications 1991 (3):199-206

34 Bailey SM, Suggett N, Walton MI and Workman P: Structure-activity relationships for DT-diaphorase reduction of hypoxic cell directed agents: indoloquinones and diaziridinyl benzoquinones. Int J Radiol Oncol Biol Phys 1992 (64):649-653

35 Walton MI, Wolf CR and Workman P: Molecular enzymology of the reductive bioactivation of hypoxic cell cytotoxins. Int J Radiat Oncol Biol Phys 1989 (16): 983-986

36 Workman P, Walton MI, Bibby MC and Double JA: In vitro response of mouse adenocarcinoma of the colon (MAC) tumours to indoloquinone EO9: correlation with bioreductive enzyme content. Br J Cancer 1990 (62):215

37 Walton MI, Bibby MC, Double JA, Plumb JA and Workman P: DT-diaphorase activity correlates with sensitivity to the indoloquinone EO9 in mouse and human colon carcinomas. Eur J Cancer 1992 (28A):1597

38 Riley R and Workman P: Enzymology of the reduction of the potent benzotriazine-di-N-oxide hypoxic cell cytotoxin SR 4233 (WIN 59075) by NAD(P)H:(quinone-acceptor) oxidoreductase (EC 1.6.99.2) purified from Walker 256 rat tumour cells. Biochem Pharmac 1992 (43):167-174

39 Hoban PR, Walton MI, Robson CN, Godden J, Stratford IJ, Workman P, Harris AL and Hickson ID: Decreased NADPH: cytochrome P-450 reductase activity and impaired drug activation in a mammalian cell line resistant to mitomycin C under aerobic but not hypoxic conditions. Cancer Res 1990 (50):4692-4697

40 Moulder JE and Rockwell S: Hypoxic fractions of solid tumours: experimental techniques, methods of analysis, and a survey of existing data. Int J Radiat Oncol Biol Phys 1985 (11):323-329

41 Vaupel P, Schlenger K, Knoop C and Hockell M: Oxygenation of human tumors: evaluation of tissue oxygen distribution in breast cancers by computerized O_2 tension measurements. Cancer Res 1991 (51):3316-3322

42 Maxwell RJ, Workman P and Griffiths JR: Demonstration of tumour-selective retention of fluorinated nitroimidazole probes by 19F magnetic resonance spectroscopy in vivo. Int J Radiat Oncol Biol Phys 1989 (16):925-929

43 Raleigh JA, Franko AJ, Treiber EO, Lunt JA and Allen PS: Covalent binding of a fluorinated 2-nitromidazole to EMT-6 tumours in BALB/c mice: detection by F-19 nuclear magnetic resonance spectroscopy at 2.35 T. Int J Radiat Oncol Biol Phys 1986 (12):1243-1245

44 Jerabek PA, Patrick TB, Kilbourn MR, Dischino DD and Welch MJ: Synthesis and biodistribution of 18F-labelled fluoronitromidazoles: potential in vivo makers of hypoxic tissue. Appl Radiat Isot 1986 (37):599-605

45 Urtasun RC, Chapman JD, Raleigh JA, Franko AJ and Koch CJ: Binding of 3H-misonidazole to solid human tumors as a measure of hypoxia. Int J Radiat Oncol Biol Phys 1986 (12):1263-1267

46 Leliveld P, Double JA, Bibby MC, Stratford IJ and Moody CJ: Antitumour activity and bioreductive potential of the mitosene GBJ 584. Annal Oncol 1992 (3, Suppl 1):101

47 Patterson LH, Maine JE, Cairns DC, Craven MR, Bennett N, Fisher GR, Ruparelia K and Giles Y: Use of N-oxides of DNA affinic anthraquinones as bioreductive prodrugs. Annal Oncol 1992 (3, Suppl 1): 94

Therapeutic Drug Monitoring and Dose Optimisation in Oncology

Merrill J. Egorin

Division of Developmental Therapeutics, University of Maryland Cancer Center and Division of Medical Oncology, Department of Medicine, University of Maryland School of Medicine, Baltimore, Maryland 21201, U.S.A.

Therapeutic drug monitoring, also frequently referred to as "clinical pharmacokinetics" or "applied pharmacokinetics", has been described as the process of using drug concentrations, pharmacokinetic principles, and pharmacodynamic criteria to optimise drug therapy in individual patients [1]. Therefore, implicit in any discussion of therapeutic drug monitoring are the consideration and integration of certain aspects of pharmacokinetics and pharmacodynamics as well as those of laboratory, clinical, and economic reality. In beginning this discussion, it is worth noting that therapeutic drug monitoring is considered standard medical practice for many classes of drugs and the practice of "applied pharmacokinetics" is gaining increasing acceptance as an intrinsic and essential part of rational drug development. Although this chapter will deal with dose optimisation in individual patients, many of the concepts and issues addressed are equally applicable to the process referred to as "pharmacologically guided dose escalation" wherein pharmacokinetic/pharmacodynamic relationships elucidated in preclinical animal studies are used as a basis to move a drug through phase I clinical trials in the most rational and expeditious fashion.

Pharmacokinetics and Pharmacodynamics

Definitions and assumptions inherent in any discussion of therapeutic drug monitoring will be addressed first. "Pharmacokinetics" may be thought of as the mathematical description of the behaviour of a drug and its metabolites in a system, whereas "pharmacodynamics" may be thought of as drug effect - both therapeutic and toxic. An often heard, and useful, rephrasing of these definitions is that "pharmacokinetics is what the body does to the drug and pharmacodynamics is what the drug does to the body." Obviously the two terms are neither the same nor interchangeable, but an inherent assumption is that they are linked. Operationally, the treatment of a patient can be conceptualised as: 1) making a diagnosis and selecting a drug; 2) administering the drug chosen, with resultant absorption, distribution, metabolism, and elimination (pharmacokinetics); and 3) observing target organ effects, both therapeutic and toxic (pharmacodynamics).

When considering the administration of a particular drug regimen, it is helpful for the clinician to visualise the potential pharmacodynamic consequences of that drug in the patient to be treated [2] (Fig. 1). This can be easily considered as a two-dimensional graph wherein intensity of drug effect is displayed along the ordinate, or vertical axis, while time, and therefore duration of drug action, is displayed along the abscissa, or horizontal axis. The utility of such an analysis is augmented if similar consideration is given to the time course of drug itself (pharmacokinetics) in the plasma, or possibly the relevant anatomic site of drug action (Fig. 1).

The relevance of pharmacokinetics to the clinical use of drugs is based on 3 experimentally verified principles which apply to many drugs [3]. First, an optimal clinical response can be obtained in most patients if drug concentration in serum is maintained

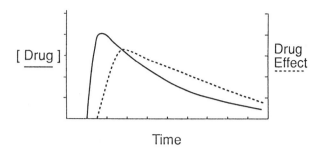

Fig. 1. Representations of time courses of a) drug effect (pharmacodynamics) and b) plasma drug concentrations (pharmacokinetics) (adapted from reference 2)

within a given range of concentrations. Second, as a result of genetic, environmental, pathophysiologic, or drug-drug interactions, there may be remarkable differences among patients in their abilities to eliminate or clear a drug from the body (interpatient pharmacokinetic variability) and in their sensitivities to a given concentration of drug (interpatient pharmacodynamic variability). Finally, as a result of these two principles, there may be wide differences among patients in the dose required to achieve an optimal clinical response. Despite this strong theoretical basis for therapeutic drug monitoring and the intuitively obvious rationale for its value, the process is not always straightforward and may have considerable limitations under certain circumstances.

Goals of Optimising Therapy for Individual Patients

The obvious goal of optimising therapy for individual patients is to maximise the proba-

bility of producing a desired therapeutic effect while minimising the probability of a toxic event occurring. With antineoplastic chemotherapeutic agents, this goal is often modified to seek the maximum likelihood of producing a desired therapeutic effect while producing acceptable toxicity. For drugs that do not produce toxicity at dosages or serum concentrations close to those required for therapeutic effects (Fig. 2a), there is little incentive for dose optimisation or individualisation. Rather, patients are treated with dosages high enough to insure achievement of therapeutic concentrations. In contrast, certain drugs, such as antineoplastic chemotherapeutic agents, which frequently produce toxicity at dosages close to those required for a therapeutic effect (Fig. 2b), provide great incentive for dose optimisation in individual patients. In practical terms, and as stated previously, successful implementation of optimal dosing strategies involves consideration of a number of pharmacokinetic/pharmacodynamic principles as well as a number of important practical issues related to patient care, sample acquisition, analytical methodology and quality assurance, and cost.

The "Therapeutic Range"

Because pharmacokinetics are known to be quite variable from one patient to another, both toxic and therapeutic responses to drug administration are frequently better correlated with plasma drug concentration, or the total amount of drug in the body, than with the dose administered. However, to use this concept, the physician needs to know the proper relationship between drug concentration in

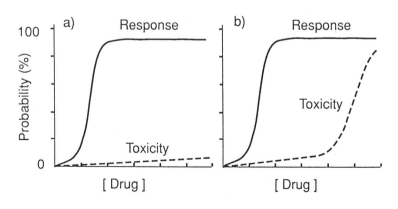

Fig. 2. Relation between drug concentration and drug effects for a hypothetical drug. a) drug with essentially no toxicity at concentrations yielding maximum probability of therapeutic response. b) drug with increasing probability of toxicity as concentrations increase above those needed for maximum probability of a therapeutic response

plasma and either the associated quantitative pharmacodynamic effect or the statistical likelihood of achieving a given toxic or therapeutic effect. Moreover, implementation of the concept may require knowing the proper relationship between concentration of drug at the site of action (e.g., tumour, bone marrow, or gastrointestinal mucosa) and at the site of sampling (e.g., plasma, saliva, urine).

The first of these issues, i.e., the relationship linking drug concentration to both toxic and desired therapeutic effects, is often referred to as the "therapeutic range" (Fig. 2b) [1]. This important term and concept can be misleading or misunderstood in a number of respects. First, the therapeutic range for most, if not all, antineoplastic agents has not even been considered, let alone defined in carefully controlled clinical trials. Second, there is no guarantee that achievement of a concentration within the so-called therapeutic range will result in a desired clinical response or that it will preclude a significant or unacceptable toxic outcome. Rather, the therapeutic range should be understood for what it is, i.e., a combination of probability charts. More specifically, it is that range of drug concentrations within which the probability of a desired clinical outcome is relatively high and the probability of an unacceptable toxicity is relatively low. However, in any individual patient, a desired clinical response might occur at what would be considered subtherapeutic drug concentrations, and conversely, toxic outcomes can occur when drug concentrations are maintained in what is considered a safe range. Furthermore, with antineoplastic agents, it is fair to assume that it is possible to achieve drug concentrations that will produce unacceptable toxicity in all patients whereas the likelihood of producing a therapeutic response may not be 100%, irrespective of how high a drug concentration is achieved. In other words, for these highly toxic substances, not only need there not be much separation in the curves relating the probabilities of therapeutic response and toxicity to drug concentration, but the maximum likelihood of achieving a therapeutic response is almost guaranteed to be less than the maximum likelihood of producing significant toxicity. Furthermore, for many drugs, there are discrete subpopulations for whom these concentration-effect relationships differ from the norm. Examples of such subpopulations include the aged, patients with poor performance status, and patients rendered abnormal due to concomitant therapy.

Unfortunately, as with the paucity of concentration-effect charts representing therapeutic ranges for antineoplastic drugs, characterisation of these extraordinary patient subpopulations is almost non-existent.

Modelling Pharmacokinetic/ Pharmacodynamic Relationships

As might be surmised from the previous discussion, there is a great need for defining the relationships between the pharmacokinetics of antineoplastic agents and their toxic and therapeutic pharmacodynamic consequences. Traditionally, modelling the *in vitro* relationship between drug concentration and effect has been based on the concept of ligands, receptors, and the relationship between occupied receptors and effect [5,6]. As a result of the hypothesis that drug effect is proportional to the fraction of receptors occupied, drug concentration-effect models have been written in terms of the law of mass action. The pictorial representation of these models is usually that of a sigmoidally shaped curve displayed on an abscissa representing drug concentration and an ordinate representing drug effect. The initial portion of such curves may show concentrations of drug which produce little or no effect, followed by a range of drug concentrations wherein drug effect increases linearly in proportion to the concentration, or logarithm of the concentration, of drug present. (Figs. 2 and 3). At still higher concentrations, as the maximum pharmacodynamic effect is approached, increasing drug concentrations produce a less than proportional or no increase in drug effect (Figs. 2 and 3). Mathematically, this *in vitro* relationship has been well described by the modified Hill equation [7-9]:

$$E = \frac{(E_{Max})(C^H)}{(C_{50}^H) + (C^H)}$$

In this equation, E_{max} represents the maximum elicitable effect, C represents concentration, and C_{50} represents that concentration

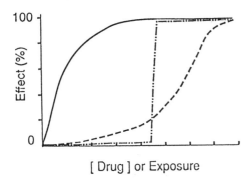

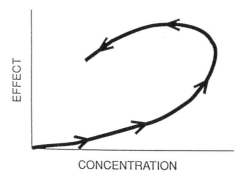

Fig. 3. Examples of relationships between concentration and effect of a theoretical drug

Fig. 4. A pharmacodynamic model displayed as a counterclockwise (reverse) hysteresis loop

which elicits 50% of E_{max}. H is Hill's constant which defines the degree of sigmoidicity of the model and allows the model to assume a variety of shapes, from a gentle hyperbola, with a negligible range of concentrations producing no effect, to a step function in which pharmacodynamic response is a virtual "all-or-none" phenomenon, going from little or no effect to E_{max} over a very narrow range of concentrations (Fig. 3).

Despite the excellent ability to model the *in vitro* relationship between drug concentration and drug effect, there is an important potential obstacle in translating such a model to *in vivo* situations, and this reflects the fact that nowhere in the Hill equation is consideration given to the element of time. No consideration is given to the fact that, for a wide variety of reasons, there is often a temporal delay between administration of drug and observation of the pharmacodynamic consequences resulting from that administration. Included among the reasons for this delay are time required for: 1) drug to be absorbed; 2) drug to be distributed to its site of action; 3) metabolism of a prodrug to one or more active metabolites; 4) signal transduction (including generation of primary and secondary messengers or translocation of drug-receptor complexes); and 5) observation of the pharmacodynamic effect if the cell or organ affected is not accessible to direct visualisation or observation. Attempts to deal with this temporal delay between drug delivery and assessment of drug effect have represented the relationship between drug concentration and effect as a counterclockwise, or reverse, hysteresis loop (Fig. 4) [4,10-13]. This model is based on the assumption that

drug effect is related to concentration of drug at the receptor, irrespective of whether that concentration occurs during a period of increasing or decreasing drug concentrations. As a result, drug effect may initially increase more slowly than do plasma drug concentrations, but then may persist or increase during the period of decreasing plasma drug concentrations, before finally returning toward baseline. In this regard, antineoplastic chemotherapeutic agents may be thought of as representing the ultimate reverse hysteresis loop. Plasma drug concentrations often increase and then decrease without any obvious associated pharmacodynamic effect such as myelosuppression, mucositis, nephrotoxicity, neurotoxicity, or antitumour response (i.e., the curve moves out and back along the abscissa with negligible vertical displacement). Subsequently, when drug concentrations are negligible, toxic or therapeutic pharmacodynamic responses are manifested, possibly going through a period when their intensity increases and then decreases (i.e., the curve moves up and then down the ordinate with no horizontal displacement).

Despite this difficulty, there has been a great deal of activity and some notable success in utilising the modified Hill equation to model antineoplastic pharmacokinetic/pharmacodynamic relationships [14-19]. This success has often reflected the substitution of the integrated area under the curve of plasma drug concentration versus time (AUC) or its surrogate, steady state plasma drug concentration (C_{ss}) during a continuous infusion of drug, for concentration in the Hill equation. The suitability of this substitution presumably reflects the fact that both AUC and its C_{ss} surrogate include the element of time.

Other models have proven useful for relating the pharmacokinetics of antineoplastic chemotherapeutic agents to their cytotoxic consequences. More than 20 years ago, it was noted that the fraction of cells surviving *in vitro* exposure to a non-cell cycle specific cytotoxic agent was well described by the relatively simple relationship:

Survival fraction= e^{-kCt},

where C represented drug concentration, t represented exposure time, and k was a constant [20,21]. This relationship has proven particularly useful for representing the clinical cytotoxic pharmacodynamic consequences of antineoplastic chemotherapeutic agents because the product of C times t is equivalent to the AUC, a clinically measurable pharmacokinetic parameter. On the other hand, the importance of time above a specific threshold concentration rather than drug exposure, as expressed as AUC, may be the critical parameter to be considered for cell cycle specific agents such as methotrexate and cytosine arabinoside. This latter issue is one which remains to be explored in clinical trials. There are an increasing number of publications in which the two models just described for relating the pharmacokinetics and pharmacodynamics of antitumour drugs have been applied to both investigational and non-investigational antitumour agents [15-18, 22-27]. For toxicities such as myelosuppression, in which the pharmacodynamic effect can be expressed as a continuous variable, percentage decrease from pretreatment platelet or leukocyte count has been related to AUC or its surrogate, C_{ss}, during a relatively prolonged continuous infusion. Similarly, there have been successful attempts at relating the pharmacokinetics of antineoplastic chemotherapeutic agents to toxicities, such as mucositis, nephrotoxicity, or neurotoxicity, which are characterised semi-quantitatively or merely as present or absent. The simplest approach to defining such relationships involves comparing (usually with a parametric test) plasma concentrations, or AUC, between toxic and non-toxic patients [28,29]. The two models described above as having proven useful for studying myelosuppression have also proven applicable to toxicities such as

mucositis. However, in these latter cases, the treated population has been stratified by AUC or C_{ss} and the percentage likelihood, or probability, of toxicity associated with a given AUC or C_{ss} has been calculated and modelled. An alternative approach that has been successfully applied to modelling the relationship between the pharmacokinetics of a drug and its associated qualitatively or semi-quantitatively assessed toxicities involves multivariate logistic regression [30-32].

There has been less work relating the therapeutic pharmacodynamic consequences of antineoplastic chemotherapeutic agents to the pharmacokinetics of those drugs. However, examples of such work have been published for teniposide [33], carboplatin [19], 5-fluorouracil [34], methotrexate [35], and 6-mercaptopurine [36]. In a number of such cases, attempts have been made to begin defining the previously mentioned concept of a therapeutic range. Modelling the relationship of therapeutic response to the pharmacokinetics of antineoplastic drugs requires certain unusual considerations. These reflect the fact that tumour shrinkage often requires several cycles of chemotherapy. Therefore, unlike toxicity in each cycle, which can be temporally related to the pharmacokinetics of agents administered in that course, tumour shrinkage often requires consideration of the pharmacokinetics of agents in multiple or successive cycles of chemotherapy. As such, attempts at relating therapeutic response to pharmacokinetics in one course of a multiple cycle chemotherapy protocol may be unduly simplistic [19]. Similarly, modelling cumulative exposure versus tumour response is also flawed due to the bias introduced by the fact that responding patients or patients without disease progression will, by definition, receive more cycles of chemotherapy, and therefore increased cumulative AUC, than will patients whose disease progresses. It may well be that the proper pharmacokinetic parameter to model versus probability of antitumour response will be exposure- or AUC-intensity, a parameter analogous to dose intensity [37], but more patient specific [38]. In this way, potential adverse effects associated with decreased AUC intensity secondary to dose reduction or treatment delay may be defined, and issues such as adverse effects of excessive toxicity due to excessive AUC may be investigated. This approach is still unexplored, and the logistics of defining drug exposure in multiple cycles of chemotherapy, often involving multiple agents, are intimidating. Therefore, implementation of such studies will require careful planning, data collection, and committment of extensive resources. Moreover, unlike end organ toxicity associated with individual agents, the relationships of pharmacokinetics and therapeutic pharmacodynamic response for a specific drug may vary from tumour type to tumour type. Finally, it is not clear which pharmacodynamic parameter will prove most appropriate for such studies. Candidates for this role include overall response rate, complete response rate, disease-free interval, time to disease progression, and survival time.

Dosing Strategies Available for Optimising Therapy in Individual Patients

Having presented the pharmacokinetic and pharmacodynamic background upon which rational dose optimisation can be implemented for individual patients, the 3 dosing strategies that can be employed can now be discussed more intelligently.

Empiric or Non-Adaptive Dosing

The simplest, least precise, and most commonly employed strategy for administering antineoplastic chemotherapeutic agents involves empiric or minimally adaptive dosing based on mean population pharmacokinetic and pharmacodynamic behaviour applied to individual patients. Some consideration may be given to the patient's height, body weight, or body surface area, but otherwise little attention is paid to patient-specific characteristics. In this regard, an agent is used at a mg/m^2 or mg/kg "dose recommended for phase II trials". This "recommended dose" is based on the results of phase I clinical trials, and its "recommendation" may involve no pharmacokinetic consideration at all.

Adaptive Dosing

The next hierarchy of dosing sophistication involves dosing strategies with adaptive input. For this approach, population studies are required to provide a data base. Generally, a regression model is used to assess the relative contribution of identifiable characteristics of patient, drug therapy, and disease state that influence plasma drug concentrations, and dosing is based on each patient's profile with regard to these characteristics. Although this approach is most successful with drugs whose clearance is closely tied to renal function, patient characteristics such as age, sex, body weight, body surface area, serum albumin, or hepatic function may be useful. The antineoplastic chemotherapeutic agent most closely identified with this approach is carboplatin [40-43], although dosing reduction strategies for methotrexate and doxorubicin have been advocated for patients with reduced renal or hepatic function, respectively [44-47]. More recently, serum albumin has been recognised as an important factor in appropriate dosing of etoposide [48,49]. The importance of pharmacogenetic differences [50,51] in rational dosing of individual patients is an area barely explored. However, Ratain and coworkers have performed an elegant series of studies showing the importance of individual patient's acetylator phenotype in determining the appropriate dose of amonafide, an investigational agent whose major route of metabolism involves acetylation [52-55]. Similarly, Lennard and co-workers have demonstrated important interpatient pharmacogenetic differences in the handling of 6-mercaptopurine and the associated pharmacokinetic/pharmacodynamic consequences of those differences [56-61].

Adaptive Control with Feedback Dosing

The most sophisticated and complex method of dosing individual patients involves input adaptive control with feedback (Fig. 5). In this approach, population-based predictive models are initially employed as above but contain provision for (and expectation of) dosing alteration, based on feedback revision of the

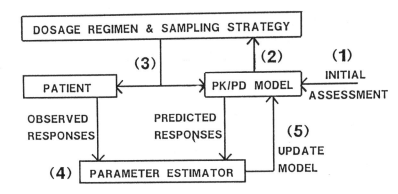

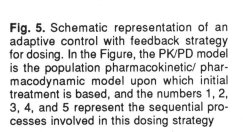

Fig. 5. Schematic representation of an adaptive control with feedback strategy for dosing. In the Figure, the PK/PD model is the population pharmacokinetic/ pharmacodynamic model upon which initial treatment is based, and the numbers 1, 2, 3, 4, and 5 represent the sequential processes involved in this dosing strategy

model following measurement of plasma drug concentrations and/or patient response. This dosing strategy reflects the reality that for most drugs a-priori dosing methods based on patient characteristics such as age, weight, body surface area, renal function, albumin, etc., may be useful for providing initial estimates of dosing needs but are usually rather imprecise because they only partially account for interpatient pharmacokinetic variability. Considerably greater precision can be obtained with predictive methods based on a characterisation of the specific drug in question in any given individual patient after an initial dose. In this fashion, plasma drug concentrations are measured at "informative" times and compared with plasma concentrations predicted by the population model with which dosing was initiated. Based on this comparison, more patient-specific pharmacokinetic parameters are calculated and dosing is adjusted accordingly to maintain or achieve the drug C_{ss} or exposure desired to produce the desired pharmacodynamic effect. If necessary, the steps of measuring plasma drug concentrations at "informative" times and comparison of those concentrations achieved with those predicted by the now hybrid patient-based/population-based model can be repeated. Based on these steps, calculation of the patient's individual pharmacokinetic characteristics can be refined further and, if necessary, additional dosing adjustments can be made. This process is most efficiently effected by combining Bayes' theorem and maximum likelihood estimation. Despite its mathematic complexity, this approach may be the only way to deliver a desired, precise exposure of an antineoplastic chemotherapeutic agent. Although this approach has been employed for several years to administer methotrexate therapy [62], more recently it

has been developed more fully and applied more widely to other investigational and non-investigational antitumour drugs [34,48,63-70]. With this increased activity, several important practical and theoretical considerations relevant to this approach to dosing have come to light.

Population Pharmacokinetic Models and Modelling

As presented earlier and outlined in the preceding paragraphs, implementation of adaptive dosing or adaptive control with feedback dosing strategies requires a model for the pharmacokinetics of the relevant agent in a population of patients [71-79]. A population pharmacokinetic model usually consists of descriptions of the modal values of important pharmacokinetic parameters, such as volume of the central compartment, volume of distribution at steady state, and total body clearance, and the variance of those parameters through the population. These values describe interpatient variability. Ideally, the quantitative importance of specific characteristics such as sex, age, change in excretory or metabolic organ function, and concomitant therapy should be included in this model. In addition to interpatient variability, the model should also address intrapatient variability by assessment of the model variance, which deals with factors such as assay imprecision and random changes in an individual patient's parameters with time. By necessity, the description of a population model is based on a sample of the entire population and this sample may or may not be representative of the whole population. This caveat needs to be considered when reviewing published population models, because small samples may give biased parameter values.

The Standard Two-Stage Approach

The population pharmacokinetic approach most commonly quoted in the literature is the standard two-stage approach. In the first stage, individual patient data sets are fitted by a variety of techniques. In the second stage, the pharmacokinetic values calculated for each patient are used to calculate the mean and standard deviation of each pharmacokinetic parameter; these means and standard deviations are considered to describe the population parameters and intersubject variability, respectively.

In theory and practice, the standard two-stage approach to defining a population model has several potential problems. While usually giving adequate descriptions of model parameters, the standard two-stage approach may overestimate intersubject variability [71,76]. Moreover, the standard two-stage approach requires "full" data sets to allow adequate performance of the non-linear curve fitting programmes with which individual patient data sets are fitted. This requirement for "full" data sets may impose the collection of between 10 and 15 blood samples with the attendant expenses incurred through personnel and assay costs. In addition, even with careful attention to detail, least squares non-linear regression analysis is often still unable to fit the data adequately and may generate clearly improbable parameter estimates for some individual data sets. This may result in discarding of those data sets when the standard two-stage approach is implemented, thereby wasting resources and potentially useful data. Alternatively, data points in individual sets, which cause problems in curve fitting, may be ignored or omitted until a fit and pharmacokinetic parameter estimates in what is felt to be "the proper range" are produced. This type of data editing has the potential of introducing unnecessary bias in the final population model produced. These drawbacks notwithstanding, the standard two-stage approach is relatively easy to implement and remains the method most com-

monly employed to describe a population pharmacokinetic model.

More Sophisticated Population Pharmacokinetic Modelling Techniques

Other approaches to the analysis of population pharmacokinetics have been developed in an attempt to address some of the potential problems associated with the standard two-stage approach. Probably the best known and most widely employed of these other approaches is non-linear mixed effects modelling, which is implemented by the computer programme NONMEM [72-78,80]. NONMEM allows the analysis of "sparse" data sets obtained in large numbers of patients to develop a description of the population pharmacokinetics. Alternative approaches [81] such as the global two-stage [82], iterative two-stage [82], and non-parametric maximum likelihood [83] analyses have also been suggested as a means to develop population pharmacokinetic models.

There have been several recent examples wherein the iterative two-stage approach has been applied to antineoplastic chemotherapeutic agents [63,64,66,67,70,84,85]. In this process, an initial population description is produced by fitting individual data sets as described for the standard two-stage approach. This description and a Bayesian algorithm are then used to refit each individual data set, and a refined population model is derived. This process of iteratively updating the population model and refitting individual data sets is continued until the population model ceases to change, although it is still unclear what specific statistical criteria define "no change". To date, application of the iterative two-stage approach to population modelling has been limited, to some extent reflecting the highly labour- and computer-intensive nature of this approach. These obstacles have been addressed, to some degree, by development of a computer programme that allows the analysis of large numbers of individual data sets and the relatively rapid completion of the multiple iterations leading to convergence and production of a final population model [86]. Although this programme and approach have recently been applied to develop population pharmacokinetic models for daunorubicin [84] and suramin [66,67,70], much theoretical work remains to be done before the relative strengths and weaknesses of this methodology are known.

There is, however, one obvious problem with the software currently available for population pharmacokinetic modelling [80,86-88], which is unfortunately, and possibly unnecessarily, computer intensive and "user unfriendly". Although the computer-intensive nature of these programmes may be inherent and thereby limit their application to centres with adequate hardware, addressing the latter of these issues should be an obvious goal for programme developers if population pharmacokinetic analyses are to be extended beyond the realm of aficionados.

LImited Sampling Strategies

A common thread in the acts of defining pharmacokinetics in individual patients, producing a population pharmacokinetic model, relating pharmacokinetics to pharmacodynamics, or adjusting dosing based on plasma drug concentrations, is the process of sampling and measuring the concentration of drug in blood (plasma, serum) or in an alternative specimen such as saliva, urine, or, possibly, tissue. The timing of such sample acquisition and analysis may be crucial to successful performance of the aforementioned tasks. Both practical and theoretical considerations exert pressure to obtain a sufficient number of samples at times that will allow the most acceptable performance of the task at hand while not resorting to sampling so excessive as to exsanguinate the patient, reduce the likelihood of the patient agreeing to treatment, or incur unnecessary work and expense for clinical personnel and the analytical laboratory. Two quite different approaches to this process of developing limited sampling strategies have been employed in clinical pharmacology studies of antineoplastic chemotherapeutic agents.

Stepwise Forward Regression

The first of these approaches to limited sampling strategy development evolved from ef-

forts to relate the pharmacokinetics and pharmacodynamics of antineoplastic drugs and was developed with the goal of estimating drug exposure, as defined by AUC, with a limited number of samples. Ratain and coworkers have employed stepwise, forward, multiple regression to produce limited sampling strategies for a variety of antineoplastic agents, including vinblastine, thiotepa, doxorubicin, cyclophosphamide, and amonafide [53,89-92]. In this approach, full, intensely sampled pharmacokinetic studies are obtained on an initial cohort of patients (the training set), and after separate univariate analyses are performed for the concentrations at each time point (independent variable) versus the AUC (dependent variable), a limited sampling strategy is developed by stepwise forward multiple regression. The F-test is used to select the optimal strategy. As a check on the forward regression analysis, data from the training set may also be subjected to stepwise, backward elimination regression analysis. Additional limited sampling strategies can be developed by initiating the stepwise regression software programme with variables other than the "best" univariate time point. The final strategy developed is then validated prospectively with a second, separate set of full pharmacokinetic profiles (the test set), correlating the estimated and actual AUC. In addition, the mean percentage of error and the mean absolute percentage of error are calculated as measures of bias and precision, respectively. The result of this exercise is an equation of the form:

$$AUC = (A \; conc_{t1} + B \; conc_{t2} + ...N \; conc_{tn}) + Z,$$

where A, B, ...N are constants which multiply the concentrations of drug measured at times t1, t2, ...tn, respectively, and Z is an additional constant which must be normalised for the dose given compared to the dose with which the limited sampling strategy was developed. This approach has the advantages of: 1) being simple to perform; 2) using inexpensive and user-friendly software; and 3) producing a relevant pharmacokinetic parameter for use in defining pharmacokinetic/pharmacodynamic relationships. Moreover, to date it has proven applicable and useful for an increasingly large number of antitumour drugs. On the other hand, the stepwise forward regression method has certain disadvantages. By definition, it only calculates one pharmacokinetic parameter, i.e., AUC or its correlate, total body clearance. Furthermore, its utility is limited to administration schedules which match that for which the strategy was developed. Therefore, a limited sampling strategy developed with a one-hour infusion would not be applicable to a pharmacokinetic study of the same drug administered by a 5-minute bolus or by a more prolonged, e.g., 6-hour, infusion. Finally, the nature of the limited sampling strategy development process and the resulting equation by which AUC is calculated make timing of sample acquisition critical. A sampling strategy requiring 1, 4, and 24-hour samples will not perform well with samples acquired at 2, 3, and 24 hours. In such cases, the expenses involved in sample acquisition, and possibly shipping and analysis, as well as patient discomfort and inconvenience are wasted because useful data cannot be derived. Furthermore, if some therapeutic intervention, such as dosage alteration, is to be based on the AUC to be calculated, patient management may be compromised.

Optimal Sampling Theory

An alternative approach to the development of limited sampling strategies, and one which has been applied successfully to studies of doxorubicin [93], involves strategies based on optimal sampling theory [94-98]. This approach is applied within a Bayesian context, and its implementation requires: 1) a pharmacokinetic model with defined, assumed, or estimated values for each parameter; 2) a random error model with parameter values; 3) an optimality criterion to be applied; 4) knowledge of the dosing regimen to be employed; and 5) a desired number of samples to be obtained and the time frame in which those samples could be obtained. In reality, this process of applying optimal sampling theory to development of limited sampling strategies is a computer-intensive process, involving software that is not particularly user-friendly. However, while more technically difficult to develop and implement than is the stepwise forward multiple regression approach, an optimal sampling theory-based limited sampling strategy results in much more flexibility. Its use in conjunction with a

Bayesian algorithm allows: 1) calculation of multiple relevant pharmacokinetic parameters, such as volume of the central compartment; 2) computer simulation of plasma drug concentration profiles after various hypothetical doses or schedules of drug administration; 3) use of samples collected at times other than those exactly specified in the limited sampling strategy. Therefore, although initially far more labour intensive than is stepwise, forward, multiple regression limited sampling strategy development, an optimal sampling theory-based limited sampling strategy should lead to less waste of economic, patient, and personnel resources. It should also provide much more flexibility in terms of developing dose optimisation strategies for individual patients. However, it must be remembered that the optimality criteria employed in developing a limited sampling strategy must be optimal for the task at hand. It may not be possible to satisfy simultaneously with common sampling times the clinical needs of: 1) assessing a drug concentration in relation to a desired therapeutic range; and 2) obtaining drug concentration measurements for use in pharmacologically-guided adaptive control with feedback dosing strategy.

Practical Considerations

In addition to the important theoretical aspects of population pharmacokinetic model development and limited sampling strategies which were just described and which will continue to be active areas of development, refinement and evolution, there are a number of very practical operational and economic factors that are inherent in an adaptive control with feedback dosing strategy [99]. These begin with drug administration where the accuracy of dosing with respect to starting time and, if parenteral dosing is employed, duration of administration should be confirmed. If oral dosing is utilised, consideration must be given to assessing time of ingestion, patient compliance with dosing schedule, and the potential for problems, such as emesis or altered diet, which could increase or decrease bioavailability. Furthermore, it must be understood that, due to patient discomfort, expense, and competition for blood for other diagnostic purposes, the number of plasma drug concentrations that can be obtained from individual patients is restricted. The impetus that this has given to development of limited sampling strategies has been discussed previously.

It should be obvious, therefore, that careful attention must be paid to obtaining those samples properly. This includes attention to the method by which, sites from which, and actual time at which samples are obtained and to collection of samples into the appropriate type of carefully labelled tube. Subsequently, care must be paid to appropriate handling of samples. This may include, if necessary, rapid separation of plasma from erythrocytes, protection from light, maintenance of reduced temperatures, and avoidance of prolonged storage among other considerations.

Adaptive control with feedback dosing may require any of a number of characteristics of the analytical chemical method employed in quantifying the drug in question. Rigorous quality assurance and control procedures must be inherent in the process. It is also likely that the analytical chemical method will need to be rapid to insure timely provision of data upon which dosage adjustment can be based. Low cost and generation of the minimum amounts of hazardous toxic chemical and radioactive waste are also likely to be desirable traits of the analysis used. Finally, provisions must be made to allow time for maintenance of the analytical instrumentation used, and back-up instrumentation must be available in case of malfunction of the primary analytical system used.

As discussed earlier, dosage adjustment based on comparison of measured versus expected plasma drug concentrations or clinical responses is usually a computer-based process. Although earlier sections of this chapter have dealt with a number of theoretical aspects of the methods and approaches used for these calculations, it is appropriate here to consider the practical aspects of implementing this process. Included among these are availability of the required software, hardware, and the personnel with the expertise to use them. Although the ideal combination of these would be an inexpensive, user-friendly programme that could be run on an affordable desktop computer, the reality is that many, if not most, available programmes are difficult for someone not exceedingly computer literate to use. Furthermore, most available software realistically requires either a fast desktop computer with a mathematics coprocessor or, better, a mini- or mainframe computer. While it may seem trivial, it should also be understood that, at some time, all personnel become ill or take vacation, and therefore, reliance on one person to process plasma drug concentration data into dosing recommendations is not a realistic or suitable situation.

Methods for Evaluating the Performance of Dose Optimisation for Individual Patients

The performance of any of the pharmacokinetically-guided dosing strategies presented earlier can, and probably should, be evaluated on 2 types of criteria [94,100].

Pharmacokinetic Criteria

The first of these utilises pharmacokinetic criteria. In this approach, the accuracy and precision of how well predicted drug concentrations compare with those actually achieved are evaluated mathematically by calculating the mean error and mean absolute error, respectively. Alternatively, accuracy and precision may be evaluated with the mean prediction error and root mean squared error, respectively [101].

Pharmacodynamic Criteria

It is important to understand that achievement of pharmacokinetic accuracy and precision does not mean that a pharmacokinetically-guided dosing strategy has achieved its desired goal. In fact, drug efficacy and toxicity can only be determined from direct clinical assessment of the patient's response to treatment. Plasma drug concentrations cannot and should not be used as the sole criteria for drug efficacy or toxicity. In reality, interpatient pharmacodynamic variability, as assessed by parameters such as the AUC_{50} described earlier, can be quantitatively as great as interpatient pharmacokinetic variability. Therefore, an ideal approach to dose optimisation of individual patients would utilise an integrated pharmacokinetic/pharmacodynamic population model and a Bayesian approach in which dosing would be initiated based on the population model but would be adjusted and made more patient specific as increased information is accrued on the individual patient's pharmacokinetic parameters and pharmacodynamic sensitivity to the agent in question. Accuracy and precision can be achieved in attaining a desired drug exposure or concentration and for each patient that desired exposure or concentration can be increased or decreased depending on their response to the drug. To date, this combined approach to antineoplastic agent administration has been most extensively developed for hexamethylene bisacetamide, an investigational differentiating agent with well characterised relationships between plasma drug concentration and acute neurotoxicities and between AUC and delayed myelosuppressive toxicities [63-65]. The experience with hexamethylene bisacetamide is currently being extended to the use of suramin, another investigational antineoplastic agent [66-70]. In view of the importance of not relying solely on achieving the desired pharmacokinetic target to assess the success of a dosing strategy, it is notable that the lack of a suitable population model relating the pharmacokinetics and pharmacodynamics of suramin has resulted in severe neurotoxicity and renal dysfunction continuing to occur despite the fact that plasma suramin concentrations can be controlled with great precision [66-70].

Cost-Value Criteria

Finally, even though pharmacokinetically guided dose optimisation for individual patients may produce the desired plasma drug concentration or exposure *and* the desired pharmacodynamic effects, it may not be useful. More specifically, the third basis by which pharmacokinetically-guided dosing can be evaluated involves formal economic analytical techniques for comparing the negative consequences (costs) and positive outcomes (effectiveness, benefits) that result from dose individualisation and optimisation [94,100, 102,103]. Put bluntly, this type of analysis asks if pharmacokinetically-guided dosing for the drug in question is worth it. Relative cost-value calculations can be done on a cost-effectiveness basis or a cost-benefit basis [101,104]. In considering these approaches, it is crucial to understand that the two types of cost-value analyses are not the same [102,103]. The two types of calculations differ in that cost-benefit analysis expresses benefit in monetary values, whereas cost-effective analysis relates the costs to some beneficial outcome without attempting to convert it to monetary gain. The choice between cost benefit-analysis and cost-effect analysis depends on the exact problem being posed and the potential for measuring benefits in monetary terms. It should be noted that the application of cost-benefit analysis to health care in general, and to drug therapy in particular, may be very difficult because it is difficult to place a monetary value on good health and to define and measure improvements objectively. To date, cost-value analysis of dose optimisation for antineoplastic chemotherapeutic agents is unreported, possibly reflecting the still early stage of development of the means to implement the dosing strategies themselves. Although not yet done, and despite potential problems, this type of analysis will be crucial if the utility of dose optimisation of various antineoplastic agents is to be evaluated intelligently.

Concluding Remarks

In summary, the successful development of antineoplastic drug to the point where it can be administered to individual patients with the precision desirable for a drug likely to have a low therapeutic index requires understanding of the information necessary for such dosing. It is only in this way that such information can be developed at the most propitious stages of the drug's development. Before initiation of phase I trials, it is helpful if there is some knowledge of the drug concentration and/or exposure required for *in vitro* activity and the conditions, such as medium and serum content, under which such determinations were made. It is also important to have an analytical chemical method for quantifying drug and, if possible, its relevant metabolites in appropriate biological matrices such as plasma, serum, urine, and possibly tissue. Phase I trials, with their broad range of doses, and resulting drug exposures and toxicities, represent the optimal point at which to: 1) produce an initial description of the population pharmacokinetic model for parent compound and, possibly, metabolites; 2) to produce initial pharmacokinetic/pharmacodynamic models for drug-induced toxicities; and 3) develop an initial limited sampling strategy. Phase II trials present the opportunity to: 1) validate and refine the limited sampling strategy; 2) refine the pharmacokinetic/pharmacodynamic models for drug-induced toxicities; and 3) begin defining the pharmacokinetic/pharmacodynamic model for therapeutic response. Phase III trials are the setting in which to: 1) continue refining the limited sampling strategy and pharmacokinetic/pharmacodynamic toxicity models resulting from phase II trials; 2) utilise the limited sampling strategy in large numbers of patients to complete definition of the pharmacokinetic/pharmacodynamic mod-el for response; and 3) combine the pharmacokinetic/pharmacodynamic models for response and toxicities in an attempt to define a "therapeutic range" for the drug. Finally, subsequent trials should evaluate dose individualisation of the agent from the standpoint of cost-benefit or cost-effect analysis so that the financial resources of individual patients and of society in general can be utilised most intelligently and effectively. It should be stressed that this framework for drug development needs to be initiated and followed despite lack of knowledge of the ultimate clinical utility of the specific drug under development. Unfortunately, by the time a drug has proven its clinical utility, it is impossible to acquire much of the information requisite in an adequate, integrated population pharmacokinetic/pharmacodynamic model upon which can be based a pharmacokinetically-guided strategy for delivering optimal doses to individual patients.

Acknowledgements

I thank Drs Nicholas Bachur and Leonard Reyno for critical reading of this manuscript and Linda Mueller and Bobbie Knickman for excellent secretarial assistance.

REFERENCES

1   Evans WE: General principles of applied pharmacokinetics. In: Evans WE, Schentag JJ and Jusko WJ (eds) Applied Pharmacokinetics, Second edition. Applied Therapeutics, Inc, Spokane WA 1986 pp 1-8

2   Peck CC, Conner DP and Murphy MG: Visualizing drug effects and drug disposition. In: Bedside Clinical Pharmacokinetics. Simple Techniques for Individualizing Drug Therapy (revised edition). Applied Therapeutics Inc, Vancouver WA 1989 pp 17-19

3   Slattery JT, Gibaldi M and Koup JR: Prediction of maintenance dose required to attain a desired drug concentration at steady-state from a single determination of concentration after an initial dose. Clin Pharmacokinet 1980 (5):377-385

4   Sadée W: Molecular mechanisms of drug action and pharmacokinetic-pharmacodynamic models. In: Borchardt RT, Repta AJ and Stella VJ (eds) Directed Drug Delivery. A Multidisciplinary Problem. Humana Press, Clifton New Jersey 1985 pp 35-49

5   Ariens EJ and Simonis AM: A molecular basis of drug action. J Pharm Pharmacol 1964 (16):137-157

6   Ariens EJ and Simonis AM: A molecular basis for drug action. The interaction of one or more drugs with different receptors. J Pharm Pharmacol 1964 (16):289-312

7   Hill AV: The possible effects of the aggregation of the molecules of haemoglobin on its dissociation curves. J Physiol (Lond) 1910 (40):iv-vii

8   Wagner JG: Kinetics of pharmacologic response. I. Proposed relationship between response and drug concentration in the intact animal and man. J Theoret Biol 1968 (20): 173-201

9   Levy G: Kinetics of pharmacologic effect. Clin Pharmacol Ther 1966 (7):362-372

10   Holford NHG and Sheiner LB: Kinetics of pharmacologic response. Pharmac Ther 1982 (16):143-166

11   Colburn WA: Simultaneous pharmacokinetic and pharmacodynamic modeling. J Pharmacokin Biopharm 1981 (9):367-388

12   Holford NHG: Drug concentration, binding and effect in vivo. Pharm Res 1984 (1):102-105

13   Bondi JV and Tanner RD: Kinetic hysteresis as a tool for analysis of pharmacokinetic data. In: Smolen VF and Ball L (eds) Controlled Drug Bioavailability. Vol. I. Drug Product Design and Performance. John Wiley and Sons, New York 1984 pp 179-202

14   Ratain MJ, Schilsky RL, Conley BA, et al: Pharmacodynamics in cancer therapy. J Clin Oncol 1990 (8):1739-1753

15   Egorin MJ, Van Echo DA, Whitacre MY, et al: Human pharmacokinetics, excretion and metabolism of the anthracycline antibiotic menogaril (7-OMEN, NSC 269148) and their correlation with clinical toxicities. Cancer Res 1986 (46):1513-1520

16   Egorin MJ, Sigman LM, Van Echo DA, et al: A Phase I clinical and pharmacokinetic study of hexamethylene bisacetamide (HMBA, NSC 95580) administered as a five-day continuous infusion. Cancer Res 1987 (47):617-623

17   Egorin MJ, Conley BA, Forrest A, et al: Phase I study and pharmacokinetics of menogaril (7-OMEN, NSC 269148) in patients with hepatic dysfunction Cancer Res 1987 (47):6104-6110

18   Trump DL, Egorin MJ, Forrest A, et al: Pharmacokinetic and pharmacodynamic analysis of 5-fluorouracil during 72 hour continuous infusion with and without dipyridamole. J Clin Oncol 1991 (in press)

19   Mortensen ME, Cacalupo AJ, Lo WD, et al: Inadvertent intrathecal injection of daunorubicin with fatal outcome. Medical and Pediatric Oncology 1991 Abstr 99 (in press)

20   Skipper HE, Schabel FM, Mellet LB, et al: Implications of biochemical, cytokinetic, pharmacologic, and toxicologic relationships in the design of optimal therapeutic schedules. Cancer Chemother Rep 1970 (54):431-450

21   Jusko WJ: Pharmacodynamics of chemotherapeutic effect: Dose-time-response relationships for phase-nonspecific agents. J Pharm Sci 1987 (60):892-895

22   Bennett CL, Sinkule JA, Schilsky RL, et al: Phase I clinical and pharmacological study of 72-hour continuous infusion of etoposide in patients with advanced cancer. Cancer Res 1987 (47):1952-1956

23   Ratain MJ, Schilsky RL, Choi KE, et al: Adaptive control of etoposide dosing: Impact of interpatient pharmacodynamic variability. Clin Pharmacol Ther 1989 (45):226-233

24   Grochow LB, Noe DA, Ettinger DS, et al: A phase I trial of trimetrexate glucuronate (NSC 352122) given every 3 weeks: Clinical pharmacology and pharmacodynamics. Cancer Chemother Pharmacol 1989 (24):314-320

25   Ackland SP, Ratain MJ, Vogelzang NJ, et al: Pharmacokinetics and pharmacodynamics of long-term continuous-infusion doxorubicin. Clin Pharmacol Ther 1989 (45):340-347

26   Schilsky RL, O'Laughlin K and Ratain MJ: Phase I clinical and pharmacological study of thymidine (NSC 21548) and cisdiamminedichloroplatinum (II) in patients with advanced cancer. Cancer Res 1986 (46):4184-4188

27   Fanucchi MP, Walsh TD, Fleisher M, et al: Phase I and clinical pharmacology study of trimetrexate administered weekly for three weeks. Cancer Res 1987 (47):3303-3308

28   Thyss A, Milano G, Renee N, et al: Clinical pharmacokinetic study of 5-FU in continuous 5-day infusions for head and neck cancer. Cancer Chemother Pharmacol 1986 (16):64-66

29   Rowinsky EK, Noe DA, Orr DW, et al: Clinical pharmacology of oral and i.v. N-methylformamide: A pharmacologic basis for lack of clinical antineoplastic activity. JNCI 1988 (80):671-678

30   Coleman CN, Halsey J, Cox RS, et al: Relationship between the neurotoxicity of the hypoxic cell radiosensitizer SR 2508 and the pharmacokinetic profile. Cancer Res 1987 (47):319-322

31   Grochow LB, Jones RJ, Brundrett RB, et al: Pharmacokinetics of busulfan: Correlation with veno-occlusive disease in patients undergoing bone marrow transplantation. Cancer Chemother Pharmacol 1990 (25):55-61

32   van Groeningen CJ, Pinedo HM, Heddes J, et al: Pharmacokinetics of 5-fluorouracil assessed with a sensitive mass spectrometric method in patients on a dose escalation schedule. Cancer Res 1988 (48):6956-6961

33   Rodman JH, Abromowitch M, Sinkule JA, et al: Clinical pharmacodynamics of continuous infusion teniposide: Systemic exposure as a determinant of response in a phase I trial. J Clin Oncol 1987 (5):1007-1014

34   Santini J, Milano G, Thyss, A, et al: 5FU therapeutic monitoring with dose adjustment leads to improved therapeutic index in head and neck cancer. Br J Cancer 1989 (59):287-290

35   Evans WE, Crom WR, Abramowitch M, et al: Clinical pharmacodynamics of high dose methotrexate in acute lymphocytic leukemia. N Engl J Med 1986 (314):471-477

36   Hayder S, Lafolie P, Bjork O, et al: 6-mercaptopurine plasma levels in children with acute lymphoblastic leukemia: Relation to relapse risk and myelotoxicity. Ther Drug Monit 1989 (11):617-622

37   Hryniuk WM: Average relative dose intensity and the impact on design of clinical trials. Sem Oncol 1987 (14):65-74

38   Evans WE: Clinical pharmacodynamics of anticancer drugs: A basis for extending the concept of dose-intensity. Blut 1988 (56):241-248

39   Greenblatt DJ: Predicting steady state serum concentrations of drugs. Ann Rev Pharmacol Toxicol 1979 (19):347-356

40   Egorin MJ, Van Echo DA, Tipping SJ, et al: Pharmacokinetics and dosage reduction of carboplatin in patients with impaired renal function. Cancer Res 1984 (44):5432-5438

41   Egorin MJ, Van Echo DA, Olman EA, et al: Prospective validation of pharmacologically based dosing scheme for the cisplatin analog, carboplatin Cancer Res 1985 (45):6502-6506

42   Calvert AH, Newell DR, Gumbrell LA, et al: Carboplatin dosage: Prospective evaluation of a simple formula based on renal function. J Clin Oncol 1989 (7):1748-1756

43   Harland SJ, Newell DR, Siddik ZH, et al: Pharmacokinetics of cis-diammine-1,1-cyclobutane dicarboxylate platinum (II) in patients with normal and impaired renal function. Cancer Res 1984 (44):1693-1697

44   Taylor SG IV, Gelman RS, Falkson G, et al: Combination chemotherapy compared to tamoxifen as initial therapy for stage IV breast cancer in elderly woman. Ann Int Med 1986 (104):455-461

45   Benjamin RS, Wiernik PH and Bachur NR: Adriamycin chemotherapy - efficacy, safety and pharmacologic basis of an intermittent single high-dosage schedule. Cancer 1974 (33):19-27

46   Brenner DE, Wiernik PH, Wesley M et al: Acute doxorubicin toxicity. Relationship to pretreatment liver function, response, and pharmacokinetics in patients with acute nonlymphocytic leukemia. Cancer 1984 (53):1042-1048

47   Sulkes A and Collins JM: Reappraisal of some dosage adjustment guidelines. Cancer Treat Rep 1987 (71):229-233

48   Ratain MJ, Mick R, Schilsky RL, et al: Pharmacologically based dosing of etoposide: A means of safely increasing dose intensity. J Clin Oncol 1991 (9):1480-1486

49   Mick R and Ratain MJ: Modeling interpatient pharmacodynamic (PD) variability of etoposide (VP-16). Proc Am Soc Clin Oncol 1991 (10):Abstr 274

50   Weinshilboum RM: Human pharmacogenetics. Fed Proc 1984 (43):2295-2297

51   Vesell ES: New directions in pharmacogenetics. Fed Proc 1984 (43):2319-2325

52   Ratain MJ, Propert K, Costanza M, et al: Population pharmacodynamic study of amonafide: CALGB 8862. Proc Am Assoc Cancer Res 1990 (31):Abstr A1074

53   Ratain MJ, Staubus AE, Schilsky RL, et al: Limited sampling models for amonafide (NSC 308847) Pharmacokinetics. Cancer Res 1988 (48):4127-4130

54   Grever MR, Staubus AE and Malspeis L. Correlation of N-acetylation phenotype with plasma levels of the N-acetylmetabolite of amonafide (NSC 308847). Proc Am Assoc Cancer Res 1990 (31):Abstr 1055

55   Ratain MJ, Mick R, Berezin F, et al: Prospective correlation of acetylator phenotype with amonafide toxicity. Proc Am Soc Clin Oncol 1991 (10):Abstr A275

56   Lennard L, Keen D, Lilleyman JS: Oral 6-mercaptopurine in childhood leukemia: Parent drug pharmacokinetics and active metabolite concentrations. Clin Pharmacol Ther 1986 (40):287-292

57   Lennard L, Van Loon JA, Lilleyman JS, et al: Thiopurine pharmacogenetics in leukemia; correlation of erythrocyte thiopurine methyltransferase activity and 6-thioguanine nucleotide concentrations. Clin Pharmacol Ther 1987 (41):18-24

58   Herber S, Lennard L, Lilleyman JS, et al: 6-mercaptopurine: Apparent lack of relation between prescribed dose and biological effect in children with leukemia. Br J Cancer 1982 (46):138-141

59   Lennard L, Rees, CA, Lilleyman JS, et al: Childhood leukemia: A relationship between intracellular 6-mercaptopurine metabolism and neutropenia. Br J Clin Pharmacol 1983 (16):359-363

60   Lennard L, Lilleyman JA: Are children with lymphoblastic leukemia given enough 6-mercaptopurine? Lancet 1987 (2):785-787

61   Lennard L, Lilleyman JS: Variable mercaptopurine metabolism and treatment outcome in childhood lymphoblastic leukemia. J Clin Oncol 1989 (7):1816-1823

62   Evans WE, Crom WR and Yalowich J: Methotrexate. In: Evans et al (eds) Applied Pharmacokinetics: Principles of Therapeutic Drug

Monitoring, 2nd edition. Applied Therapeutics Inc, Spokane WA 1986 pp 1009-1056

63 Conley BA, Forrest A, Egorin MJ, et al: Phase I trial employing adaptive control dosing of hexamethylene bisacetamide (HMBA, NSC 95580). Cancer Res 1989 (44):3436-3440

64 Conley BA, Forrest A, Egorin M, Zuhowski E, et al: Adaptive control phase I trial of hexamethylene bisacetamide (HMBA) with and without concurrent alkalinization. Proc Am Soc Clin Oncol 1988 (7):61

65 Forrest A, Conley BA, Egorin MJ, et al: Adaptive control of hexamethylene bisacetamide (HMBA) pharmacodynamics. Proc Am Soc Clin Oncol 1988 (7):61

66 Scher HI, Jodrell DI, Iversen JM, et al: The use of adaptive control with feedback to individualize suramin dosing. Cancer Res 1991 (in press)

67 Jodrell D, Zuhowski E, Egorin M, et al: Intermittent bolus dosing with suramin: The use of adaptive control with feedback (ACF). Proc Am Soc Clin Oncol 1991 (10):92

68 Hutson R, Arzoomanian R, Tombes MB, et al: Test dose guided rapid iv suramin infusions with weekly iv maintenance doses. Proc Am Soc Clin Oncol 1991 (10):99

69 Cooper M, LaRocca R, Stein R, et al: Pharmacokinetic monitoring is necessary for the safe use of suramin as an anticancer drug. Proc Am Assoc Cancer Res 1989 (30):963

70 Iversen J, Scher H, Motzer R, et al: Suramin (SUR): Impact of individualized pharmacokinetics (PK) dosing on outcome in patients with prostatic cancer (PC) and renal cell carcinoma (RCC). Proc Am Soc Clin Oncol 1991 (10):103

71 Grasela TH Jr, Antal EJ, Townsen RJ, et al: An evaluation of population pharmacokinetics in therapeutic trials. Part I. Comparison of methodologies. Clin Pharm Therap 1986 (39):605-612

72 Sheiner LB, Rosenberg B and Marathe VV: Estimation of population characteristics of pharmacokinetic parameters from routine clinical data. J Pharmacokinet Biopharm 1977 (5):445-479

73 Sheiner LB and Beal SL: Evaluation of methods for estimating population pharmacokinetic parameters. I. Michaelis-Menten model: routine clinical pharmacokinetic data. J Pharmacokinet Biopharm 1980 (8):553-571

74 Sheiner LB and Beal SL: Evaluation of methods for estimating population pharmacokinetic parameters. II. Biexponential model and experimental pharmacokinetic data. J Pharmacokinet Biopharm 1981 (9):635-651

75 Sheiner LB and Beal SL: Evaluation of methods for estimating population pharmacokinetic parameters. III. Monoexponential model: routine clinical data. J Pharmacokinet Biopharm 1983 (11):303-319

76 Sheiner LB: The population approach to pharmacokinetic data analysis: Rationale and standard data analysis methods. Drug Metabolism Rev 1984 (15):153-171

77 Beal SL: Population pharmacokinetic data and parameter estimation based on their first two statistical moments. Drug Metabolism Rev 1984 (15):173-193

78 Beal SL and Sheiner LB: Estimating population kinetics. CRC Critical Rev Biomed Engin 1982 (8):195-222

79 Whiting B, Kelman AW and Grevel J: Population pharmacokinetics theory and clinical application. Clin Pharmacokin 1986 (11):387-401

80 Beal SL and Sheiner LB: The NONMEM system. Am Statistician 1980 (34):118-119

81 Steimer JL, Mallet A, Golmard JL, et al: Alternative approaches to estimation of population pharmacokinetic parameters: comparison with the nonlinear mixed-effect model. Drug Metabolism Rev 1984 (15):265-292

82 Prévost G: Estimation of a normal probability density function from samples measured with non-negligible and non-constant dispersion. Internal Report, Anders-Gerbios. 2 avenue du ler mai, F-91120 Palaiseau. 1977

83 Steimer JL, Mallet A and Mentré F: Estimating interindividual pharmacokinetic variability. In: Rowland M, Sheiner LG and Steiner JL (eds) Variability in Drug Therapy, Description, Estimation and Control. Raven Press, New York 1985 pp 65-111

84 de Valeriola D, Forrest A, Egorin M, et al: Standard (S2S) vs Iterative (IT2S) 2 stage population analysis of daunorubicin (D1) and daunorubicinol (D2) pharmacokinetics. Proc Am Assoc Cancer Res. 1991 (32)178

85 Jodrell D, Forrest A, Hawtof, J, et al: The population pharmacokinetics of CI941, a novel anthrapyrazole anticancer agent. Clin Pharm Therap 1991 (49):195

86 Forrest A, Hawtof J and Egorin MJ: Evaluation of a new program for population PK/PD analysis - Applied to simulated phase I data. Clin Pharm Therap 1991 (49):153

87 D'Argenio DZ and Schumitzky A: ADAPT II user's guide. Biomed Simulation Resources USC, Los Angeles 1990

88 D'Argenio DZ and Schumitzky A: A program package for simulation and parameter estimation in pharmacokinetic systems. Comp Prog Biomed 1979 (9):115-134

89 Ratain MJ and Vogelzang NJ: Limited sampling model for vinblastine pharmacokinetics. Cancer Treat Rep 1987 (71):935-939

90 Ackland SP, Choi KE, Ratain MJ, et al: Human plasma cyclophosphamides of thiotepa following administration of high-dose thiotepa and cyclophosphamide. J Clin Oncol 1988 (6):1192-1196

91 Ratain MJ, Robert J and van der Vijgh WJ: Limited sampling models for doxorubicin pharmacokinetics. J Clin Oncol 1991 (9):871-876

92 Egorin MJ, Forrest A, Belani CP, et al: A limited sampling strategy for cyclophosphamide pharmacokinetics. Proc Am Soc Clin Oncol 1989 (8):63

93 Launay MC, Milano G, Iliadis A, et al: A limited sampling procedure for estimating adriamycin pharmacokinetics in cancer patients. Br J Cancer 1989 (60):89-92

94 Peck CC and Rodman JH: Analysis of clinical pharmacokinetic data for individualizing drug dosage regimens. In: Evans WE, Schentag JJ and Jusko WJ (eds) Applied Pharmacokinetics. Second edition. Applied Therapeutics Inc, Spokane WA 1986 pp 55-82

95 D'Argenio DZ: Optimal sampling times for pharmacokinetic experiments. J Pharmacokinet Biopharm 1981 (9):739-756

96 Schumacher GE: Choosing optimal sampling times for therapeutic drug monitoring. Clin Pharm 1985 (4):84-92

97 Lacey L and Dumme A: The design of pharmacokinetic experiments for model discrimination. J Pharmacokinet Biopharm 1984 (12):351-365

98 Peck CC and Perkins SW: Optimal sampling theory in a Bayesian context: a framework for choosing number and timing of clinical drug level measurements. Clin Pharmacol Ther 1984 (35):26

99 Jusko WJ: Guideline for collection and analysis of pharmacokinetic data. In: Evans WE, Schentag JJ and Jusko WJ (eds) Applied Pharmacokinetics. Second edition. Applied Therapeutics Inc, Spokane WA 1986 pp 9-54

100 Voeh S: Cost-effectiveness of therapeutic drug monitoring. Clin Pharmacokin 1987 (13):131-140

101 Sheiner LB and Beal SL: Some suggestions for measuring predictive performance. J Pharmacokin Biopharm 1981 (9):503-512

102 Dao TD: Cost-benefit and cost-effectiveness analysis of drug therapy. Am J Hosp Pharm 1985 (42):791-802

103 Doubilet P, Weinstein MC and McNeil BJ: Use and misuse of the term "cost effective" in medicine. New Engl J Med 1986 (314):253-255

Current Strategies in Anticancer Drug Discovery Within the EORTC

G. Schwartsmann

EORTC New Drug Development Office, Free University Hospital, De Boelelaan 1117, 1081 HV Amsterdam, The Netherlands

Advances in the treatment of malignant diseases have been limited by our failure to identify unique biochemical and/or biological properties which are able to clearly distinguish cancer cells from the normal cell population. Consequently, currently available anticancer agents lack tumour selectivity and possess a narrow therapeutic index [1].

The great majority of anticancer agents in clinical use exert their effects through the inhibition of cell proliferation (Table 1). For instance, alkylating agents (e.g., cyclophosphamide) and antitumour antibiotics (e.g., doxorubicin) interact directly with DNA, antimetabolites (e.g., cytarabine or methotrexate) block key enzymes in the synthesis of DNA and/or RNA precursors, while tubulin-interacting agents (e.g., vincristine) interfere with the function of the mitotic spindle apparatus.

Traditional approaches for anticancer drug discovery have been largely empirical. Large-scale random screening of natural products and chemicals has been performed by the US National Cancer Institute (NCI) for over 4 decades, resulting in the identification of about half of the agents presently available for routine use [2]. However, most agents identified via the NCI screening programme were shown to exhibit significant antitumour effects against only a limited number of rapidly growing malignancies in man, such as acute leukaemias, lymphomas and certain paediatric cancers. In fact, marked advances were observed in the management of the above diseases, with a significant percentage of patients achieving a prolonged disease-free survival and, in some cases, curability. Unfortunately, the impact of cytotoxic therapy in the outcome of the most frequent solid tumours of the adult, such as colorectal, lung and breast cancer, remains very limited [3].

Recent advances in the study of molecular and cellular biology of cancer have enabled us to identify novel biochemical targets for the treatment of malignancy, such as oncogenes, growth factors, signal transduction proteins and other specific proteins involved in the malignant process. In this chapter, the EORTC anticancer drug discovery strategies will be reviewed. Special emphasis will be given to the re-evaluation of our current approach for random screening and, more important, to the possible ways to incorporate new insights on tumour biology into our future strategies for rational drug development.

Table 1. Conventional targets in anticancer therapy

Target	Examples
DNA	alkylating agents intercalators
DNA/RNA synthesis	antimetabolites DNA polymerase inhibitors
Mitotic spindle	vinca alkaloids
Hormone receptors	anti-oestrogens

Adapted from Schilsky, ASCO Educational Symposia, 1991

The Discovery of Current Anticancer Agents

A significant number of clinically active anticancer agents were discovered as a result of random screening of natural products and synthetic chemicals in rodent tumours, in some cases following preliminary observation of their antiproliferative effects in specific tumour systems (Table 2). Plant extracts (e.g., vinca alkaloids and, more recently, taxol) and microbial fermentation broths (e.g., doxorubicin, mitomycin C and bleomycin) are examples.

Rational application of scientific advances in the field of biochemistry and cancer biology was crucial for the development of antimetabolites such as 5-fluorouracil, thioguanine or cytarabine. The synthesis of antifolates such as methotrexate by Farber and colleagues followed their initial observation of a stimulatory effect of folates on the growth of human leukaemia, illustrating very clearly the importance of the association of scientific observation and rational chemical synthesis.

Table 2. Strategies for the discovery of standard cytotoxics

Strategy	Examples
Screening of natural products	vincristine doxorubicin bleomycin mitomycin C
Screening of synthetic chemicals	thiotepa busulfan carmustine mitoxantrone
Targeted synthesis	methotrexate cytarabine 5-fluorouracil thioguanine
Analogue synthesis	cyclophosphamide etoposide chlorambucil carboplatin
Rational/serendipity	mechlorethamine asparaginase mitotane cisplatin

Adapted from ref. 2

The development of hormonal agents such as tamoxifen and flutamide are the result of efforts in rational chemical synthesis. This approach has also contributed to the development of analogues of known agents, usually as a result of the rational exploitation of potential advantages in terms of antitumour spectrum, pattern of toxicity or pharmaceutical properties over the parent compounds. Cyclophosphamide, melphalan, ifosfamide, etoposide and, more recently, carboplatin are examples of the success of this approach.

The careful observation of tissue specificity in the biological activity of certain compounds also represented a valuable tool for the discovery of new anticancer agents. Examples of this approach are the demonstration of the antitumour effects of asparaginase in acute lymphoblastic leukaemias, mitotane in adrenocortical carcinomas, meta-iodo-benzylguanidine (MIBG) in neuroendocrine tumours and, more recently, suramin in adrenal and prostatic cancer [4].

Perhaps the best illustration of the combination of serendipity and rational application of scientific knowledge in anticancer drug development has been the discovery and development of cisplatin. While studying the effect of electric fields on the growth of *E. coli*, Rosenberg and co-workers observed that an alternating current passing through platinum electrodes generated various metal complexes that caused elongation and inhibition of cell growth. This finding stimulated the evaluation of the antitumour potential of platinum complexes in experimental tumours, leading to the identification of cisplatin as a highly active compound both in murine and human tumour models. Later on, its marked clinical activity was demonstrated in a variety of human tumours such as germ-cell tumours and ovarian cancer [5].

The Original NCI *In-Vivo* Compound-Oriented Screening Programme

Since 1955, a large-scale programme of random drug screening has been conducted through the NCI. This was considered the largest and most important programme for random screening of new anticancer agents available worldwide. Drug selection was based mainly on the *in vivo* pre-evaluation of new compounds in highly sensitive, rapidly growing murine leukaemias, such as the L1210 leukaemia, and latterly on the P-388 leukaemia alone. Active compounds in the pre-screen were then evaluated in a panel of murine solid tumours and human tumour xenografts (Table 3) [6].

One of the main conceptual problems with the above approach to anticancer drug screening was the observation that experimental tumours often exhibited very high sensitivity to cytotoxic agents and, as a rule, the performance of compounds in this model did not reflect adequately the behaviour of solid tumours occurring in man. In the clinic, solid tumours display marked heterogeneity of behaviour and drug sensitivity, and high resistance to cytotoxic therapy.

Furthermore, the leukaemia pre-screen tumours were usually inoculated in the peritoneal cavity, with the experimental agent being administered via the same route. Again, this approach did not reflect the situation in the clinic, where cytotoxic agents are mostly given to the patients by an intravenous injection through a peripheral vein, implying that the agent has to cross various physiological barriers before reaching the tumour site. With the intraperitoneal tumours, the cells see a very high exposure to the drug.

Another limiting factor was the observation that solid tumours growing in the patient double much slower than experimental tumours implanted in mice. In addition, the number of tumour cells inoculated in experimental animals was usually small, in comparison with the estimated tumour burden present at the time of clinical diagnosis. Thus, by the time patients received treatment, the expected number of resistant tumour cells was in general much higher than in the experimental models.

It is important to emphasise, however, that the use of the murine leukaemia pre-screens was very effective in directing drug development towards the discovery of active agents against rapidly growing human malignancies, such as leukaemias and lymphomas. However, it would be unrealistic to expect that a system based on that pre-screen would have the power to identify compounds with

Table 3. NCI compound-oriented *in-vivo* tumour panel

Pre-screen in P388 leukaemia ip/ip
↓
Panel for evaluation of antitumour activity

Murine tumours	Human tumour xenografts
L1210 ip	LX-1 sc
B-16 ip	CX-1 sc
Lewis lung ip	MX-1 sc
C-38 sc	MX-1 src (later)
CD8F1 sc	
M5076 ip (later)	

---

ip=intraperitoneal; sc=subcutaneous; src=sub-renal capsule; activity= 25% increase in life-span

great cytotoxic potential against solid tumours in the clinic. For that reason, the NCI panel was later modified, with the inclusion of additional solid tumour lines of murine and human origin. However, the initial evaluation followed essentially the same strategy, i.e., the use of the P388 leukaemia as a pre-screen.

The New NCI *In-Vitro* Disease-Oriented Screening Programme

Since its creation, over 600,000 compounds were screened for antitumour activity through the NCI. However, only a few agents showed activity against common solid tumours in the clinic. Therefore, in 1985, a new strategy was implemented for the random screening of new compounds. By this new approach, an *in-vitro* panel was created, including about 60 different tumour cell lines of human origin and representing the various common solid malignancies. The concept behind this approach was that a disease-oriented tumour panel might have a better chance to identify new compounds showing preferential cytotoxicity against certain cancer types, such as common solid tumours. In order to enable the evaluation of a large number of compounds in such a complex *in-vitro* panel, a high throughput rapid colorimetric method, initially using the MTT dye reduction and later on the SRB protein assay, was utilised [7].

AVERAGED TGI   MEAN GRAPH OF NSC 332598

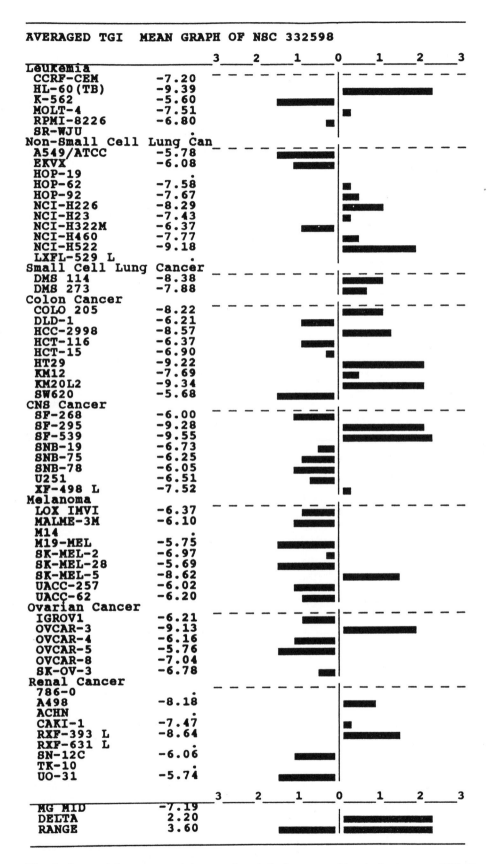

Fig. 1. Cytotoxicity pattern of the novel antitubulin agent rhizoxin in the new NCI disease-oriented screening panel. The horizontal bars indicate the relative activity of the drug in the different human tumour lines.

This approach has already produced provocative findings. By comparing cytotoxicity profiles of compounds tested in the panel, a preliminay basis for the selection of candidates for further evaluation was established. The selection could be made by the uniqueness of the cytotoxicity pattern in the panel or a more specific antitumour activity against certain clusters of tumour cell lines.

Notably, structurally unrelated compounds having a common intracellular target could be identified by means of their common cytotoxicity profiles in the screen. For example, the cytotoxicity profile of the experimental tubulin-interacting agent rhizoxin is very similar to that observed for other structurally unrelated tubulin binders, such as vincristine, vinblastine or taxol (Fig. 1). The profile of topoisomerase II inhibitors such as etoposide also showed a high correlation coefficient with other structurally unrelated topoisomerase II inhibitors such as doxorubicin or mitoxanthrone [8].

In order to exploit optimally the information generated by the new NCI screen, efforts are necessary to characterise the tumour cell lines included in the panel, with regard to their biochemical and biological properties. This could be of great value for the correct interpretation of the results obtained in the screen. In addition, it may allow us to address mechanistic questions which can guide us in the selection of promising compounds for further testing.

However, there are obvious limitations to this in-vitro screening programme. The observation of cytotoxic effects of a specific compound in the panel does not necessarily mean that the effects will be translated into efficacy in the in-vivo situation. Animal studies, especially in human tumour xenografts, will remain necessary to evaluate the pharmacodynamic behaviour of the candidate compound. Similarly, the panel would in principle fail to identify agents that need metabolic activation, such as cyclophosphamide or ifosfamide. Furthermore, agents acting through the immune system, or via the interaction with other tissue components, such as the stroma, will certainly be missed by the screen.

The EORTC New Drug Discovery Programme

In order to establish a comprehensive European programme for anticancer drug development, the EORTC New Drug Development Coordinating Committee (NDDCC) was created in 1981. This committee includes representatives of the EORTC preclinical and clinical groups, as well as experts from the U.S. National Cancer Institute, the U.K. Cancer Research Campaign and the German Cancer Society. The main objective of the NDDCC is to improve the speed and efficiency of anticancer drug development within the EORTC.

The aims of the NDDCC are executed by the New Drug Development Office (NDDO), which was created in 1984 and is located at the Free University Hospital and the Netherlands Cancer Institute in Amsterdam, The Netherlands. The NDDO is responsible for the acquisition of new compounds, coordination of preclinical screening programmes, drug formulation and synthesis, animal toxicology studies and the coordination and monitoring of phase I and II clinical trials [9].

Until now, new compounds, without prior systematic evaluation, have been submitted to the screening programme developed by Fiebig et. al. at the University of Freiburg in Germany [12]. By contrast, new agents with prior in-vitro or in-vivo evaluation and/or a clear scientific rationale are channelled through the various EORTC preclinical groups for further testing. Compounds are evaluated mainly by the Clonogenic Assay Screening Study Group (CASSG), the Screening and Pharmacology Group (SPG) and the Pharmacology and Molecular Mechanisms Group (PAMM). These groups are composed of chemists, cell biologists, pharmacists, pharmacologists, toxicologists and clinicians who have high expertise in the in-vitro and in-vivo evaluation of experimental cytotoxic agents.

The evaluation of a new compound through the EORTC Preclinical Groups includes not only the determination of antitumour activity, but also the definition of therapeutic index. The combination of in-vitro and in-vivo antitumour activity studies, preclinical pharmacokinetics and animal toxicology studies are very important in the assessment of the potential therapeutic index of new candidate compounds. For instance, transplantable mouse colon adenocarcinomas (MAC tumours), which are generally refractory to cytotoxic agents, have been utilised for the evaluation of the antitumour effects of new candidate compounds in comparison with their toxicity to bone marrow cells. Preclinical studies of flavone acetic acid and, more recently, the evaluation of a series of ether lipids and tubulin-interacting agents have followed the above-mentioned strategy [10].

The Screening Programme at the University of Freiburg

In this screening programme new compounds are evaluated in a 4-step system including in-vitro and in-vivo studies. The first step consists of the in-vitro evaluation of the compound in a panel of human solid tumour cell lines propagated as human tumour xenografts (HTX) subcutaneously in the nude mouse. Cytotoxicity tests are initially performed in 6 tumour cell lines, selected on the basis of their sensitivity to standard anticancer agents, i.e., a very sensitive non-small cell lung carcinoma line, 2 moderately sensitive small cell lung and breast carcinoma lines, and 3 resistant melanoma, colorectal and ovarian carcinoma lines (Table 4).

Table 4. Drug screening programme - University of Freiburg

In vitro testing of 6 HTX

    NSCLC
    SCLC
    Breast
    Melanoma
    Colon
    Ovary

In vivo testing of sensitive* HTX sc

Extended *in vitro* testing in HTX/human bone marrow

Extended *in vivo* testing of sensitive HTX sc

---

* Selection made on the basis of antitumour profile as well as 50% inhibitory concentrations (IC50)

Compounds showing significant antitumour activity at this stage (based on the percentage of responding lines and/or drug concentrations needed for a target cytotoxic effect), are then tested in vivo in the same tumour cell lines exhibiting sensitivity during the in-vitro steps [11]. If sufficient activity is confirmed in vivo, additional in-vitro and in-vivo tests are performed, including the estimation of the potential therapeutic index of the compound (tumour versus human bone marrow cells).

A significant potential advantage of HTX models for anticancer screening is the high prediction rate for both resistance and sensitivity of a tumour. Retrospective studies utilising standard cytotoxic agents suggest a predictive value for clinical resistance of about 90%, while the prediction for clinical activity is around 50-60%. Furthermore, experiments are highly reproducible, the pharmacodynamic behaviour of the compound can be evaluated in vivo, and the model is also suitable for combination chemotherapy studies [12].

The main limitations of the utilisation of the HTX model are the high costs, the need for special laboratory facilities, and the logistical problems of setting up a large-scale in-vivo testing facility. Nevertheless, it appears to be the best available system for the secondary evaluation of potentially interesting new compounds identified through in-vitro primary screening methods.

Preclinical Phase II Studies Using the HTX Model

Considering the large number of negative phase II clinical trials performed within the framework of the EORTC during recent years, and the preliminary observation of a high correlation between the antitumour activity of standard anticancer agents in the HTX model and their clinical outcome, a prospective multicentre study to evaluate the potential use of this model to pre-select candidate compounds for clinical trials was activated under the sponsorship of the NDDO.

The selection of tumour lines to be included in the testing panel was performed from a large pool of those available at various participating European centres. As a result, 4-8 HTX per tumour type, differing in histology, growth rate and chemosensitivity, were chosen. These represented the most frequent solid tumour types encountered in the clinic, such as breast, colorectal, melanoma, ovary, head and neck and non-small cell and small cell lung carcinoma.

Four agents, 2 of them representing one active (doxorubicin) and one inactive (amsacrine) drug in solid tumours in the clinic, as well as 2 experimental agents in clinical development, were selected in the first phase of the study. Preliminary results with the above-mentioned strategy have indicated its feasibility on a multicentre basis, and have confirmed the efficacy of doxorubicin and the inactivity of amsacrine in the panel. At present, a second phase of the study is ongoing, whereby cisplatin and diaziquone or AZQ are being tested as prototypes of active and inactive agents in the clinic [13].

Promising Agents Deriving from Standard Approaches

Taxol and Taxotere

Taxol is a plant alkaloid isolated from the bark of the Pacific yew, *Taxus brevifolia*, having emerged through the process of random screening at the NCI. In contrast to the vinca alkaloids, which inhibit microtubule assembly, taxol promotes microtubule assembly and stabilisation. This agent has shown impressive activity in initial clinical trials, including ovarian and breast cancer, melanoma and leukaemias [14]. Further clinical evaluation of taxol has been hampered by supply problems, which hopefully will be solved by alternative routes of extraction and/or chemical synthesis. Taxotere, a semisynthetic analogue of taxol, has been found to be equally active in preclinical models and is completing phase I clinical trials in Europe. The main toxicities of these agents during initial clinical trials were myelosuppression, mucositis, peripheral neuropathy and allergic reactions. By early 1992, the NDDO will coordinate a broad phase II evaluation of taxotere in patients with solid tumours.

Topotecan and CPT-11

Topoisomerases I and II are nuclear enzymes which function by relaxing supercoiled DNA. They act as catalysts for the passage of DNA strands through single and double-strand breaks, by nicking and rejoining.

Topoisomerase inhibitors form stable enzyme-DNA cleavable complexes, leading to lethal DNA strand breaks [15]. During cell division, topoisomerase II cleaves both strands of the DNA helix, forming a protein bridge with DNA until continuity is re-established. Epipodophyllotoxins such as etoposide, and intercalating agents like doxorubicin are potent inhibitors of topoisomerase II.

Topoisomerase I also takes part in the process of breakage and resealing of DNA, but is only capable of cleaving single DNA strands. Acridine-related intercalators and dactinomycin are able to stabilise the topoisomerase I-DNA complex, but camptothecin was until recently the only example of a specific topoisomerase I inhibitor evaluated in human trials. Unfortunately, initial studies of this compound revealed only moderate antitumour activity, but unpredictable bone marrow toxicity and life-threatening haemorragic cystitis [16].

Considering that topoisomerase I inhibitors are expected not to be cross-resistant with topoisomerase II inhibitors, considerable interest in the clinical evaluation of camptothecin analogues was generated. Topotecan and CPT-11 are 2 newly developed camptothecin analogues, which are undergoing clinical evaluation. Both agents have shown significant antitumour activity during initial phase I trials. Objective tumour responses to topotecan were documented during phase I trials mainly in patients with lung cancer, while phase I and II trials of CPT-11 revealed antitumour activity mostly in lung, colorectal and gynaecological malignancies. The main dose-limiting toxicities of these compounds are to the bone marrow and gastro-intestinal tract. Both will be evaluated in phase II trials in patients with colorectal and lung cancer within the framework of the NDDO.

Anthrapyrazoles

The anthrapyrazoles are DNA intercalators structurally related to mitoxanthrone, which have gained considerable attention during the last few years. Preclinical studies with one of the compounds of the series, CI-941, revealed impressive antitumour effects. Notably, preclinical studies were performed mainly in murine tumour models. Recently, CI-941 completed phase II trial in patients with advanced breast cancer, showing objective responses in about 60% of the patients [17]. It is an example of a compound with considerable interest for further development.

Suramin

Suramin has been used for decades against trypanosomiasis and other parasitic diseases. Clinical studies with this polysulphonated naphthylurea were initially performed in AIDS patients, following the observation of anti-viral properties of the compound in vitro. However, antitumour activity was observed in a patient with AIDS-related non-Hodgkin lymphoma. Also, adrenal insufficiency was documented during exposure to the compound. Consequently, clinical studies were initiated in other tumour types, including lymphoma, adrenocortical carcinoma, and prostatic cancer [18]. Although the mechanism of action of this agent is not yet fully elucidated, suramin possesses a variety of effects on signal transduction, cell adhesion and migration, and growth factor-receptor interactions. It inhibits glycosaminoglycan metabolism and has effects on heparin-binding growth factors and angiogenesis factors.

The main toxicities of suramin in early clinical trials were coagulopathy, proteinuria, creatinine elevation, bone marrow suppression, adrenal insufficiency and neuropathy. However, the most severe complication observed so far with this agent was the development of a Guillain-Barre-type neuropathy, which is more frequent in patients exposed to serum drug levels in excess of 300 µg/ml. Considering that antitumour activity was ob-

served in vitro at serum levels around 200 µg/ml, monitoring of drug concentrations is essential. The compound has a prolonged serum half-life of about 21 days and is extensively protein-bound. Drug elimination appears to depend mainly on renal excretion, and no significant drug metabolism has been documented [19].

Moving Towards Rational Development

Recent advances in the understanding of tumour cell biology have stimulated the NDDCC and NDDO to direct their drug discovery programme towards rational development. These advances have revealed a series of potential new avenues in anticancer therapy (Table 5). Therefore, current efforts will concentrate on the acquisition of compounds that may interact with novel cellular targets.

Agents such as those acting at the tumour cell membrane level or influencing the function of membrane constituents, such as adhesion molecules and proteolytic enzymes, are of great interest. Similarly, compounds interfering with signal transduction proteins such as novel ether lipid analogues are already in evaluation in animal models through the NDDO. In addition, new protein kinase C inhibitors related to staurosporin will soon initiate in-vitro testing within the framework of the EORTC. Other interesting compounds for evaluation are growth factor inhibitors (such as EGF, TGF, PDGF antagonists) and oncogene blockers including antisense oligonucleotides [20]. Other chapters in this monograph deal with the possibilities and present limitations in the development of antisense oligonucleotides and membrane/signalling drugs.

The evaluation of agents that circumvent drug resistance is also considered a priority. At present, 2 compounds that appear to interfere with P-glycoprotein function are under evaluation by the NDDO. The non-immunosuppressive cyclosporin analogue PSC833 will soon start phase I evaluation through the EORTC Early Clinical Trials Group (ECTG), while the calcium antagonist flunarizine is

Table 5. Potential new targets in anticancer therapy

Cell membrane/constituents

Growth factors and receptors

Signal transduction proteins

Oncogenes

Cell cycle regulatory genes/proteins

Extrachromosomal DNA

Hypoxia

Tumour cell differentiation

Tumour vasculature

Topoisomerase I*

Mitochondria*

Microtubules*

---

* Conventional intracellular targets recently exploited by new promising experimental anticancer agents
Adapted from Schilsky, ASCO Educational Symposia, 1991

completing its preclinical evaluation. However, there are still important methodological limitations in the clinical evaluation of these compounds to be overcome [21].
The clinical testing of agents that induce tumour cell differentiation, such as retinoids and vitamin D analogues, represents another exciting area for future development. By this approach, the balance between cancer cell proliferation and differentiation is restored, due to the induction of maturation and a consequent decrease in the proliferative capacity of the tumour. This strategy has been successfully tested in various preclinical models, including acute promyelocytic leukaemia, neuroblastomas and germ-cell tumours, and initial clinical trials with differentiation inducers such as retinoic acid and hexamethyl bisacetamide (HMBA) are ongoing [22].
The pathophysiology of tumour-related angiogenesis is still to be understood. The ability of certain tumours to form new blood vessels which support the neoplastic growth appears to be dependent on the production of certain polypeptides which possess angiogenic properties. Therefore, the search for inhibitors of tumour angiogenesis represents

another fascinating area for future studies [23].
Similarly, hypoxia has been recently recognised as a potential tool for the development of a more selective form of anticancer therapy. Bioreductive alkylating agents are activated to more cytotoxic metabolites under hypoxic conditions, which may provide a physiological means of preferential cell kill in poorly vascularised solid tumours. The bioreductive indoloquinone EO9, which will soon start clinical trials through the NDDO, is the prototype of a compound exploiting this approach, being at least 10 times more cytotoxic against tumour cell lines *in vitro* under hypoxic conditions. EO9 is bioactivated by the enzyme DT-diaphorase and may exhibit particularly good activity against tumours rich in this enzyme [24].

Concluding Remarks

A superficial appreciation of the achievements of the last 4 decades in the field of anticancer drug development might give the false impression that little has been accomplished in the treatment of malignancies, especially with respect to curability of the common solid tumours of the adult. However, it is important to recognise that oncology is a new speciality and, in contrast to other areas of medicine, covers a large number of individual diseases, each of them highly heterogenous in behaviour. Furthermore, anticancer drug discovery efforts so far have been largely based on empiricism, because detailed information on tumour biology and the cellular and clinical pharmacology of anticancer agents always lagged behind their application in the clinical setting.
In spite of the fact that we have failed to discover any form of "cancer-specific" therapy, major improvements in the outcome of less frequent tumour types, such as acute childhood leukaemias and Hodgkin's disease, have occurred. Nevertheless, success was never an easy task to be accomplished, even in the above context. In fact, the advances that led to curability of these types of cancer did not derive exclusively from the identification of new active agents, but followed a long

and stepwise learning process about the natural history and patterns of failure in these diseases, the proper handling of cytotoxic agents in combination, and the recognition of the importance of a multidisciplinary treatment approach.

It is very important that scientists involved in anticancer drug discovery programmes retain a broad view of the potential strategies to be exploited. It is undisputable that recent advances in cancer biology have disclosed new and fascinating avenues in drug development, which should be of high priority in our future programmes. However, various agents showing interesting activity in recent trials, such as taxol, topoisomerase I inhibitors and the anthrapyrazoles, are derived from so-called "traditional" methods for drug screening.

Therefore, it may be also possible that, by the identification of new active cytotoxic agents exhibiting favourable toxicity profiles, cure will be achieved in refractory solid tumours by means of conventional drug combination strategies. So it can be argued that, as long as the reasons for tumour sensitivity or resistance to the drugs are addressed, a certain amount of random screening of new compounds should remain as an alternative approach to be pursued by the NDDO, especially considering the diversity of chemical structures and mechanisms to be expected from compounds derived from natural sources. Therefore, considering the scale and sophistication of the NCI *in-vitro* screen, new compounds acquired by the NDDO will be submitted routinely to that panel for primary evaluation. Also, it is our commitment to assist the NCI in the better characterisation of their tumour cell lines. Those agents considered of interest for further evaluation by the EORTC will undergo their secondary screening in individual disease-oriented panels of HTX representing common tumours in the clinic.

In summary, novelty of chemical structure and mechanism of action, a broad or unique spectrum of antitumour effects in preclinical models, and a clear scientific rationale are considered the key features for the selection of new compounds for further development through the NDDO. Similar criteria are also in use by the Cancer Research Campaign Phase I/II Clinical Trials Committee in the UK and there is extensive collaboration with them. As a challenge for the near future, our main task should be to take the enormous amount of information recently derived from cancer biology forward into new strategies for rational development.

REFERENCES

1   Schwartsmann G, Winograd B and Pinedo HM: The main steps in the development of anticancer agents. Radiotherapy and Oncology 1988 (12):301-313

2   Sikic BI: Anticancer drug discovery. JNCI 1991 (83):738-740

3   Corbett TH, Valeriote FA and Baker LH: Is the P388 murine tumor no longer adequate as a drug discovery model? Invest New Drugs 1987 (5):3-20

4   Garaventa A, Guerra P, Arrighini A, et al: Treatment of advanced neuroblastoma with I-131- meta-iodobenzylguanidine. Cancer 1991 (67):922-928

5   Rosenberg B: Fundamental studies with cisplatin. Cancer 1985 (55):2303-2316

6   DeVita VT, Oliverio UT, Muggia FM, et al: The drug development and clinical trials program of the Division of Cancer Treatment, National Cancer Institute. Cancer Clin Trials 1979 (2):195-217

7   Skehan P, Storeng R, Scudiero D, et al: New colorimetric cytotoxicity assay for anticancer drug screening. JNCI 1990 (82):1107-1112

8   Paull KD, Shoemaker RH, Hodes L, et al: Display and analysis of patterns of differential activity of drugs against human tumor cell lines: development of mean graph and COMPARE algorithm. JNCI 1989 (81):1088-1092

9   Schwartsmann G, Wanders J, Koier I, et al. EORTC New Drug Development Office coordinating and monitoring programme for phase I and II trials with new anticancer agents. Eur J Cancer 1991 (27):1162-1168

10   Double JA and Bibby MC: Therapeutic index: a vital component in the selection of anticancer agents for clinical trial. J Natl Cancer Inst 1989 (13):988-991

11   Berger DP, Fiebig HH, Winterhalter BR, et al: Preclinical phase II study of ifosfamide in human tumor xenografts in vivo. Cancer Chemother Pharmacol 1990 (26):S7-S11

12   Fiebig HH, Berger DP: Characterization of a human tumor xenograft panel for preclinical drug development and studies on tumor biology. In: HH Fiebig, DP Berger (eds) Immunodeficient Mice in Oncology. Karger Verlag, Basel, in press

13   Boven E, Winograd B, Fodstad O, et al: Preclinical phase II studies in human tumor lines: a European multicenter study. Eur J Cancer 1988 (24):567-571

14   Rowinsky EK, Cazenave LA, Donehower RC, et al. Taxol: a novel investigational antimicrotubule agent. JNCI 1990 (82):1247-1259

15   Hsiang YH, Hertzberg R, Hecht S, et al. Camptothecin induces protein-linked DNA breaks via mammalian DNA topoisomerase I. J Biol Chem 1985 (260):14873-14878

16   Ohno R, Okada K, Masaoka T, et al. An early phase II study of CPT-11: a new derivative of camptothecin for the treatment of leukemia and lymphoma. J Clin Oncol 1990 (8):1907-1912

17   Pinedo HM and Schwartsmann G. New drugs. In: Powles TJ and Smith IE (eds) Medical Management of Breast Cancer. Martin Dunitz 1991 pp 167-176

18   Stein CA, LaRocca RV, Thomas R, et al: Suramin: an anticancer drug with a unique mechanism of action. J Clin Oncol l989 (7):499-508

19   LaRocca R, Stein C, Myers C, et al: Suramin induced acute polyneuropathy. Proc AACR 1989 (8):71

20   Reed JC, Stein C, Subasinghe C, et al: Antisense mediated inhibition of BCL2 protooncogene expression and leukemia cell growth and survival: comparison of phosphodiester and phosphorothioate oligodeoxynucleotides. Cancer Res 1990 (50):6565-6570

21   D'Incalci M, Broxterman HJ and van Kalken CK: Membrane transport in multidrug resistance, development and disease. Ann Oncol 1991 (20):635-639

22   Breitman TR and Sherman MI: In vio model systems for differentiation therapy of leukemia and solid tumors. In: Waxman S, Rossi GB, Takau F (eds) The Status of Differentiation Therapy of Cancer. Raven Press, New York 1988 pp 263-275

23   Folkman J, Weisz PB, Jouille MM, et al: Control of angiogenesis with synthetic heparin substitutes. Science 1989 (243):1490-1493

24   Walton MI, Smith PJ and Workman P: The role of NAD(P)H: quinone reductase (EC 1.6.99.2,DT-Diaphorase) in the reductive bioactivation of the novel indoloquinone antitumor agent EO9. Cancer Communications 1991 (3):199-206